OUT
of the
NORM

OTHER BOOKS BY AUTHOR:

Lower middle grade (ages 6-12)
THE ADVENTURES OF ROSIE HART SERIES:
    Fairy Quest
    Mermaid Rescue
    Unicorn Mission
    Dragon Hunt

Picture books
LITTLE MONSTER'S BOOK OF FEELINGS (available in English, Czech and English/Czech bilingual version)
THE ADVENTURES OF A CHOCOLATE BUNNY

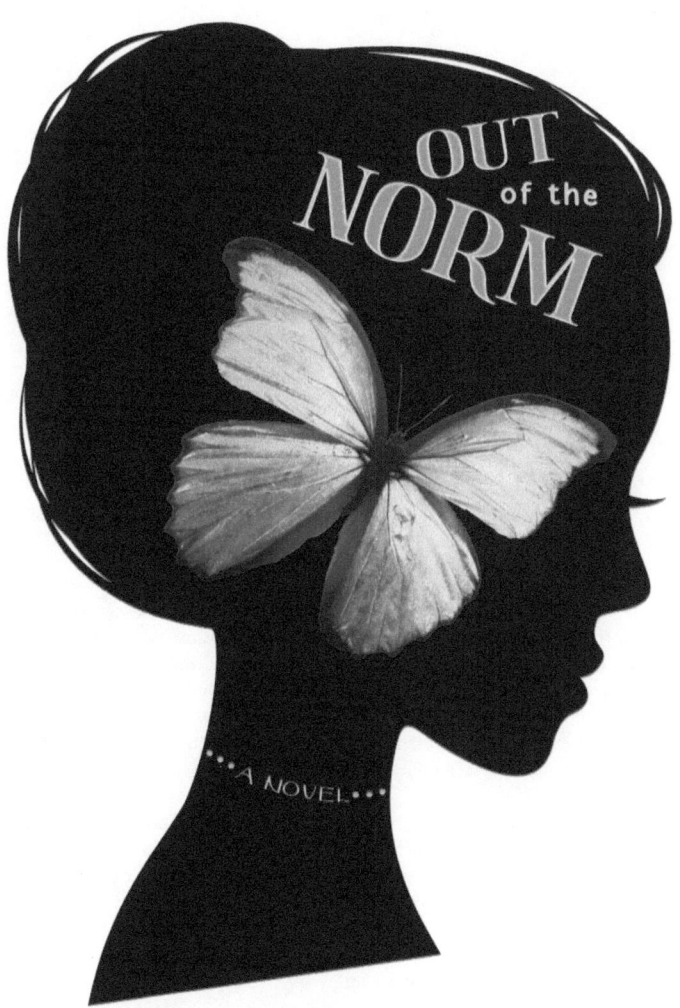

This book is dedicated to all women
who have ever struggled to achieve their dream.

A catalogue record for this book is available from the National Library of New Zealand.

Copyright © 2023 by Iveta Ongley. ALL RIGHTS RESERVED.

This book is a copyright. Except for the purpose of fair review, no part may be stored or transmitted in any form or by any means, electronic or mechanical, including recording or storage in any information retrieval system, without permission in writing from the publisher/author. No reproduction may be made, whether by photocopying or by any other means, unless a licence has been obtained from the publisher/author, except in the case of brief quotations in critical articles or reviews.

This book is a work of fiction. Names, characters, businesses, organizations, places, events and incidents either are the product of the author's imagination or are used fictitiously. Any resemblance to actual persons, living or dead, events, or locales is entirely coincidental.

For more information, or to book an event, contact:
Iveta Ongley - iveta@ivetaongley.com
ivetaongley.com

ISBN 978-1-7385809-4-1 (paperback), 978-1-7385809-8-9 (hardcover), 978-1-7385809-5-8 (e-book)

First Edition: July 2023

JOIN MY NEWSLETTER

Do you want to keep in touch with my world of writing and be the first to know about new releases, sales, and events?

Then scan the QR code and sign up to my newsletter.

As a thank you gift, you'll receive a FREE pdf download of *My Journey to Motherhood companion* (paperback and hardcover versions are also available for purchase).

My Journey to Motherhood companion is a book of poems, prompts and journalling pages for women struggling with pregnancy, divided into six sections, Dreaming, Miscarriage, Pregnancy, Birth, Holding you, and Pleasures of Motherhood. It contains a poem, 20 journalling prompts and 20 journalling pages for each section.

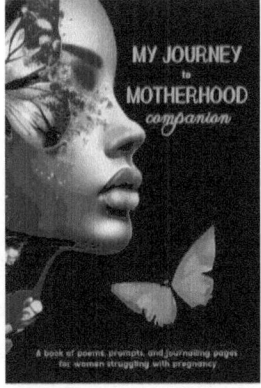

NOTES ON CONTENT

While this novel is a work of fiction, it is based on my experiences and medical struggles during my own pregnancy journey. In no way do I recommend women struggling with similar issues to follow the medical advice given in this book. It is important to always consult a medical professional for all health-related needs.

This book contains adult scenes and language and is suitable for readers aged 18+.

Trigger warning: on-page sexual assault, miscarriage, and birth

CHAPTER 1

"We regret to inform you that after a thorough examination, your application has been declined."

Anita's eyes filled with tears, blurring her vision. Still, she continued staring at the screen, reading the email.

"We have determined that you do not meet the eligibility criteria for our programme."

The world around her dimmed. It was as if someone had covered the sun, leaving her in the dark, with only the bright computer screen blazing in front of her. The future she had imagined, the future where she became a mother, had disappeared. Anger bubbled in her stomach, making its way into her mind.

What requirements did I fail? I have a safe home, a good job, and enough money in my bank account to last me until the end of my life. I don't take drugs and don't smoke and drink only occasionally, but who doesn't? It would definitely be quite hard to find a woman who doesn't like the odd glass of wine or two. I certainly don't know any. How hard would it be to just write what they actually didn't like? Too hard, obviously.

"We would like to assure you that our decision was based solely on medical criteria and does not reflect any personal opinions or judgments about your character or circumstances."

"Bollocks! What complete bollocks!" Anita screamed.

My doctor has absolutely no concerns about my health and I lead a good lifestyle. But I know what their issue is. It can't be anything else. And it will be the same issue that the previous three agencies declined me for. I'm sure of it. Well, I thought I was living in the 21st century, but it feels like I've stepped back in time. How can they be so prejudiced? So, I don't have a partner. So what? I'm a single woman wanting to have a baby. Do they really put so much weight on my status? I'm perfectly capable of bringing up a child on my own. If I had a partner, I wouldn't need to approach them, right? Duh. How ridiculous.

Anita didn't want to cry, but the weight of the bad news overwhelmed her, and at that moment, she lacked the will to hold her tears back. She stifled a sob before letting the grief take control of her, and then cried until her heart and soul dried the last tear off. She didn't know how long she had cried, allowing her body to deal with the situation. Even with an exhausted body and a sore head, her mind raced with thoughts and emotions.

Screw them all. I won't beg anyone anymore. No, I'm done with this rubbish. It is my right as a woman to bring a baby into this world. Who are they to tell me I'm not a suitable candidate because I don't have a partner? They should know that women who approach them do it as the last resort. But they don't care, do they? ... Of course, I would much rather find a nice man who I could have a child with. If only I could. If only my body allowed me to do so. Seeing a handsome man turns me on, but he just can't come anywhere near me. I just can't help that I hate being touched, that even the thought of it flips my stomach upside down. It's not like that I can change who I am, is it? And getting pregnant without a man touching me is virtually impossible. But they don't know that, do they? They just judge me based on their stupid criteria. They don't understand how hard it is living without touch. I don't mind when the children at work need a cuddle or when friends give me a hug, that's alright. But when a man tries to touch me sexually, my body betrays me. What am I going to do? What the hell am I going to do? ... But I need to do something. I can't give up now. No, I won't let them stop me. Nobody has the right to tell me I can't have a baby. Nobody. If the clinics won't give me sperm, I will have to get it myself. Somewhere. Somehow. Even if it means the torture of having sex.

Shivers ran down Anita's spine and cold sweat trickled down her back. Her entire body shuddered, but she had to overcome this. There was no other way. If she ever wanted to become a mother, she simply had to.

Ok, she thought with determination, *I need a plan; a brilliant plan. ... First, the timing will have to be perfect. There's no room for mistakes. I'll have to do it when I'm ovulating to give my body the highest chance of becoming pregnant. And also, to lessen the number of times I'll have to have sex.* Anita shuddered again. *Good thing I know my body rhythms well,* she continued planning, trying to push the disturbing thoughts away. *Thank goodness for the first clinic telling me to start recording my body changes. I can't believe that it has been almost a year. All the time I had wasted with these so-called women's support agencies and clinics. Well, I'm done with them now. Anyway, I'm the one who will be laughing at the end. I'm a pro now at taking my basal temperature and studying the changes in my discharge and cycle. And so I know exactly when I'm ovulating. Getting the time right will be a piece of cake.*

The place has to be perfect too. Where should I go? I can't have a one-night stand in Maidenhead. That just wouldn't work, oh no. In our little town, everyone knows everyone. And if the person I hooked up with didn't know me, one of their friends would. Nah, that would be a complete disaster. The whole town would soon know what happened and the one thing I'm sure about is that I don't want anyone to know who the father of the child is. Nope, this baby will be mine and mine only, and no man will be involved in bringing it up.

I'll have to go out of town, that's clear. But where? Reading? Or maybe Windsor? Slough? No, neither would do. They are all too small, just like Maidenhead, and way too close to home. I'm sure that I would come across someone who knows me there too. No, the only possible solution; the only city big enough is London. Nobody knows me there and I don't know anyone either. And I bet it will be pretty easy to go to a nightclub or a bar and find a man willing to have a no-questions-asked sex.

Now Anita had reached her decision, a great weight settled in her heart. With her mind clear on what she had to do but her guts squirming in disgust, she was truly torn. Having a vision, a plan of what she needed to do, was great, but she hated what she had to do for it. Her decision was filling her with dread, but she had no other option than to betray herself; to betray her senses and emotions, to betray her soul. She knew she would have to repeat the trip several times. Getting pregnant straight away would be amazing, but Anita didn't believe she would be that lucky. The premise of having to do it several times spun her head and brought the bitter taste of stomach juices into her mouth.

DING DONG! rang the bell at the door, interrupting Anita's agonising brainstorm. She jumped and ran to the door, her heart racing.

"Hello, are you ready for our shopping trip?" Anita's best

friend, Zara, chirped. "Oh Anita, what happened?" she exclaimed, noticing Anita's red, puffy eyes and shaky composure.

"I received another rejection letter," Anita admitted, after ushering Zara into the house.

"Oh, hunny. I'm so sorry," said Zara, hugging Anita.

Anita melted into the comforting hug, sobbing.

"It will be ok. I promise. You will have a baby one day. I'm sure you will."

"I'm done with these agencies. All the questions and weird looks I get when I stride in on my own. I just want a baby and they keep on telling me I'm not suitable. Screw them all. They don't want to help me? Then be it. Who needs them, anyway? I'll get a baby by myself!" cried Anita, wetting Zara's shoulder with her tears.

"That's the spirit. Yes, I'm sure we could find a nice man willing to be the donor. Chris might even know someone. Do you want me to ask him?"

Chris was Zara's fiancée. And no, Anita didn't want Chris and Zara searching for a man for her.

Anita pulled away from Zara. "I don't want you to find me a man. I know you mean well, but I don't want a man in my life. All I want is a baby. And I don't want anyone to know who the father is and for the father to be involved. Like at all!"

"But hun, it would be good. He could help with the upbringing, give you a break sometimes, you know? And, he would pay you child support," Zara winked.

A spark of anger ignited inside Anita. "I don't need money Zara. Mum and Dad left me the house and enough money to live comfortably, you know they did. The wage I get from the nursery is a bonus. I don't need a sugar daddy. This will be my baby. Only mine."

Anita's pulse raced. She knew she shouldn't shout at Zara, her wonderful, loyal Zara who had stood by her side through all the good and bad. But all the regret and disappointment gathered inside her over the last year drowned her other thoughts. A gate had opened and all the hurt and pain gushed out. And unfortunately, Zara was at the receiving end.

"Ok, if that's what you want. I'm just trying to help," whispered Zara, backing away.

Anita unclenched her fists, her pulse slowing down, her anger subsiding to nothing, and tears trickling down her cheeks again.

"I'm so sorry, Zara. I'm so sorry. I shouldn't have shouted at you. None of this is your fault. You are the last person I want to be angry at. I'm just so sick of everything and everyone."

"I know you are. It must be extremely hard. I'm sure that I would be very stressed if I were in your situation. Well, now, tell me how you are planning to get pregnant then." Zara asked.

Anita's eyes flicked from her friend's face to the floor and back. She knew Zara wouldn't agree with her idea. She was still in two minds about it herself.

"Well, I have decided," Anita mumbled, "to go to London and have a one-night stand."

Zara's eyes popped out of her head. "Are you serious? That's so dangerous! And stupid! And did I say dangerous? You can't do that. Anything could happen. You could get hurt."

"It won't be so bad. People do it all the time."

Anita picked up the kettle to make a cup of tea to stop her hands from shaking.

"Yes, and people get hurt all the time, too. You hear it on the news and read it in the newspapers. Anita, I won't let you do it!"

Anita slammed the kettle on the counter, her mind racing. "Zara, you have no right to tell me what to do. I have made my decision. Next time I'm ovulating, which is next week actually, I'll be heading to London to get pregnant."

Anita glared at her best friend, her body shaking. How she hated Zara at that moment for bringing these things up. Deep inside, she knew how dangerous and stupid her plan was, but so far, she had kept these troubling thoughts hidden. Now they were out and she couldn't put them back.

"I'm sorry, Anita. I know this is your decision. I just don't want you to get hurt. I'll come with you, ok?"

Anita grumbled, "I don't want you to come with me. It's going to be embarrassing enough without you looking over my shoulder."

"Well," said Zara, laughing. "I wouldn't be looking over your shoulder during the actual act, would I? That would just be weird."

"You know what I mean," said Anita. "I need to go alone. Please, let me do it alone. I know you don't agree, but I have to try. I've got nothing else left. If I don't give this a go, I might always wonder if it could have worked."

Anita watched Zara purse her lips.

"You are correct. I don't agree with this idea at all. I still think it's too dangerous and you shouldn't do it. But ... I know you'll do it anyway, Anita. You are too stubborn to give up, and you have wanted a baby for too long. You were right, it's not my place to forbid you to do it, but can you promise me that you'll be very careful? And you'll message me every half an hour you're out. I don't care if it takes the whole night. I won't go to sleep until you are back home. I want to know you're safe. Can you do that?"

Anita hugged Zara tight. The hate she had felt a minute earlier turned to pure love. She loved this woman more than anyone in the world. They had been best friends since kindergarten and had shared all their ups and downs together. Zara held her up when Anita's parents died in a car crash. Anita wouldn't have survived that ordeal without her. Zara pulled her out of the deep pit she had fallen in and taught her how to live again. Anita didn't eat or drink, she didn't want to talk, she didn't want to live. Every second of her life was too much; every moment too painful to go on. It had taken several long months for Anita to start seeing the light again and to gain some will to push through. She couldn't believe it had been ten years already. How she missed her mum at that moment; tears pricked her eyes again as her heart ached for the embrace she could never have.

"Shall we go shopping now? You will need a new dress for your wild night out," grinned Zara.

Anita heard the insincere tone in her voice; she knew Zara too well. But at least she was on board, and that was enough.

"Yes, let's go," Anita agreed, happy for the mood to lighten up. "Let me grab my bag."

CHAPTER 2

The music blasted so loud Anita could hardly think. The entire room resonated with the song's deep bass; even the ground felt like it was moving to the rhythm. A crowd of bodies swayed on the dance floor, with a strobe light flashing above their heads, creating a vision of still black and white images. The air smelled of sweat and alcohol, a weird combination which, in some sense, worked.

Anita dashed into the bathroom, aware of each heartbeat in her chest, which seemed to be in perfect sync with the bass blaring in her ears. Despite her best efforts to relax, she was tense and ready to flee at the first opportunity. Checking her face and dress in the mirror, she tried to get her act together, but the sense of dread wouldn't disappear. She was more nervous than before her first date. Anita didn't like physical contact but, understandably, as a teenager experimented a bit. She had a few boyfriends in her past, but the relationships never continued for long. When the boys tried to touch her, a sense of disgust would spread through her body. And the unbearable ordeal of sex was just too much for her, so she gave up, committing to life without touch.

Anita closed her eyes, focusing on her goal, on the future she had dreamed of having. She imagined herself holding a baby, the baby clutching her finger and softly cooing. The tightness in her body eased and her heartbeat slowed down a little. The illusion was working, but the calmness she had aimed for didn't come. Far from it. Sighing, she gave her whole appearance one last glance, and walked into the loud and crowded venue. Once at the bar, Anita ordered a ginger beer and turned around, glancing at the sea of faces. A few men had already given her a nod on her way to the bar, raising their drinks in a greeting.

I'm like a horse at a parade, she chuckled.

A tall blond man sitting at the bar nearby turned to look at her. Their eyes met, and he made a move.

"Hi there. How are you tonight?" he began with the typical opening line.

Not very original, thought Anita, but aloud she said, "Hello, I'm good."

"I don't think I've seen you here before."

"This is my first time. I don't usually come to this club, but I needed a change of scenery."

Anita sipped the beer, avoiding eye contact. She was so out of her element, unsure how to navigate this unfamiliar territory of flirting. She didn't want to share her true identity with anyone there, but she had to up her game. Quickly making up a fake name, she said, "I'm Stella."

"Nice to meet you, Stella. Thomas. So, why did you need a change of scenery?" he asked.

"Well, you know how it is. The places you go to all the time get boring. The same people, the same music, the same mood. I wanted something new, something more exciting tonight," Anita said, trying to sound mysterious and flirty while her sweaty hands clutched the bottle tight.

Surely, he must have noticed her shaky voice and composure, but it looked like he didn't. He was oblivious to how she felt. Instead, his interest heightened.

He turned towards her and in a deeper voice said, "I know of an exciting place if you want to come."

"I'm all game tonight," said Anita, an icy stream trickling down her back. "Let me run to the ladies first."

Anita rushed to the bathroom, collapsing in the cubicle, her nerves as tight as a wire and her fingers stiff from holding the beer bottle. She stretched her frozen knuckles, surprised that the bottle withstood her firm grip. Anita's vision spun, and her breathing faltered.

What am I doing? What the hell am I doing? This is so wrong. I don't want to do this. She straightened up, regaining some of her composure. *I'm not doing this. I'm going home. I've been so stupid! Why did I even think that I could do this?*

Anita sent a quick message to Zara.

> I've chickened out. Going home

> Good, message me when you get back

With stealthy ninja-like moves, Anita stuck her head out of the bathroom. A few people gave her a funny look, but she couldn't care less. Scanning the area, she ducked into the crowd and, weaving through the partying people, made her way to the door. Once outside, she sped towards the nearest Tube station, anxiety squeezing her chest. The further she ran, the calmer her mind was. But the calmer she was, the slower her body moved. And when the cool night air had cleared her mind completely, she stopped.

Where do you think you are going, Anita? You can't run away like this. It will always be the same. You need to go back and finish what you have started. You can't leave now. ... Oh, come on Anita. You can do this. You have to do this. You've dreamed of having a baby for so long. Don't give up now. You can't give up on your dream. Come on, you silly goose! Turn around and go back! That's right, turn around and walk back towards the club. There you go. You're doing it. Well done. And here you are. Now, go inside and find Thomas. Good.

As if in a dream, she found Thomas still sitting at the bar.

"Oh, here you are. Are you ready?"

"Yep. Where are we going?" said Anita, hoping the confident demeanour wouldn't betray her true emotional state.

"A friend of mine is having a party. It will be exciting, I promise," he winked at her.

Anita trembled, but she followed Thomas out of the club. They talked about nothing in particular, the small talk suiting Anita just fine. She was a complete mess on the inside. Her heart had settled up in her throat, and mind buzzed in panic. The only thing that kept her going was the dream of having a baby. Her own little baby.

Soon, the river came into view. They headed towards a brightly lit boat tied to the pier. Music and laughter blasted from the boat, with several groups of people mingling on the main deck.

"Thomas! You made it!" a short, dark-haired man shouted. "And who would this be?" he motioned towards Anita with an approving nod.

"This is Stella. Stella, meet Jake."

"It's lovely to meet you for sure," Jake continued. "Come in, come in, both of you. Make yourselves at home. Thomas, you know where things are. I'll come and see you soon," he said before rushing off.

"Care for a drink? Jake's got everything imaginable here. He loves parties."

"Does he live on the boat?"

"Oh yes, he's a bit of an adventurer. He lives on it, works on it and parties on it even more."

Thomas chortled, enjoying his own joke.

Anita felt like vomiting. She'd had enough of the experience already. She knew she had to speed things up if she didn't want to spend the entire night there.

"Yes, please. A glass of red will be perfect. And maybe we could talk somewhere quieter," she suggested, gazing straight into Thomas's eyes in what she hoped was at least a bit seductive.

Thomas gasped. "Sounds good."

He ran to the bar, grabbed two glasses and a bottle of wine, and led the way down the stairs to a little cabin under the main deck.

"Come in. Here should be quiet enough."

Anita walked into a cosy room with two sofas and a table. She could still hear the party raging above them, but the room was reasonably quiet. She put her bag on one sofa while Thomas opened the wine. Pouring them both a glass, he passed her one.

"Cheers."

"Cheers." Anita let the wine trickle down her throat, hoping it would calm her nerves a little.

A shot of something stronger would have been better, she thought.

Her eyes on Thomas, she put the glass on the table.

Thomas came near. She lifted her head, her entire body shivering as he leaned in for a kiss. Anita's heart skipped a beat. She dreaded this moment. She could barely manage touching, so having someone's tongue in her mouth was next level sickening. His warm breath reached her lips, causing the tingle of nausea to return.

I can do this. I can do this. I can! ... No, I can't. I'm going to be sick. Oh no, he's pulling me closer now. God, I can't bear his touch; I can't bear his lips. He needs to stop. I'd hoped it would be ok, that it wouldn't be as bad as I remember. I'd hoped that somehow things would be different this time, better in some way. But they're not. They're as horrendous as before. I feel so sick. ... Ouch, my ears are so sore, it feels like my heart is going to jump out of them. The goosebumps all over my body feel like a grater and I must look like I got an electric shock with all my hair standing up. How is he not noticing it? How is he not noticing any of this? Does he think I am so excited or what? Yes! He does, obviously! He's trying to undress me now. The zipper is giving him a lot of trouble. Oh my goodness, how long does it take to unzip a dress? How long is this going to take? Come on, Anita. If you are going through with this, do something too. He needs to think you want the same. You've gone too far to stop now.

Anita pulled Thomas's T-shirt off. Palms sweating and hands shaking, she was grateful for no buttons to fuss with. Thomas unzipped his pants and let them fall down. Their underwear and shoes joined the pile on the floor. Anita had never been so exposed, so vulnerable. Thomas sat down on the sofa, leading Anita on top of him. When he entered her, Anita almost threw up. Swallowing hard several times to get rid of the sick taste in her mouth, she tried to regain her composure.

If only he stopped breathing into my face. It stinks. It must be the wine. But what else? There is a hint of something else. It's so awfully warm, absolutely disgusting. I can't do this. ... Yes, I can. And I will. I have to, now. I cannot stop in the middle. Is he done yet? How long will this take? Oh no, now he wants to lie down.

Thomas lifted Anita up and laid her on the sofa. Lowering his body on top of her, he pushed his penis harder and harder inside her. His hands caressing her skin burnt like fire. His chest rubbing against her chest scratched her breasts. Anita struggled to hold back screams; her entire body being torn apart from the inside out. Desperate for this to end, she faked squeals of ecstasy to speed things up, letting out some of the pain and disgust she had been feeling. She clung to the hope that her ordeal would soon end. And then it was finally over. Thomas gave one last powerful thrust, followed by a deep grunt, before collapsing on top of her.

Thank goodness he's done. Anita held her tears back, her spirit raw and broken. Crying at that moment wouldn't do. *Just get off me now. Get off!*

As if reading her mind, he rolled onto the sofa beside her, panting.

"Well, this was quite exciting, wasn't it?" he said, visibly pleased with himself and his performance. The tone of his voice turned Anita's stomach over again. She hated this smutty small talk afterwards almost as much as she hated the act itself.

Forcing a smile, she said, "It certainly was."

Happy with the answer, he leaned over and passed her the wine. Anita accepted the glass; she needed something to wash the revolting taste from her mouth. What she needed even more was a long hot shower to wash him and the sweat off her body. She could still feel his touch, she could still smell his smell, and it made her dizzy. The whole room smelled of sex.

However, what Anita needed the most was to get away.

The universe must have listened to her wish, because at that very moment her handbag started vibrating. Anita almost tripped to get to it, her heart rejoicing on hearing Zara's voice.

"Anita! Are you ok? Are you back home?"

"Yes, I'm ok. I'm sorry I haven't messaged you. No, I'm not home."

"You're not home? Where are you? What are you doing?"

"Not now," said Anita, her brain working fast. "I cannot come right now."

"What are you talking about?"

"I'm busy. I cannot come and help you right now," Anita repeated, willing Zara to understand.

To her relief, she did.

"Yes, you have to. I need you."

"It will have to wait."

"No, it can't wait. I need you here now! I need you here NOW!" Zara shouted.

Anita pulled the phone away from her ear to protect her drum. Surely, Thomas would have heard the last sentence.

"Ok," Anita moaned, pretending to be disappointed. "I'll come."

She turned to Thomas. "I'm so sorry. My sister suffers from occasional night terrors, and I'm the only one who can calm her down. I'll have to go."

"Ok. I understand."

Anita gathered her clothes and shoes, her body trembling. She needed to pee, but not here, not now. Barely zipping her dress up, she rushed up to the deck, tripping on the steps in her high heels. *Stupid shoes.* She darted off the boat, wanting to disappear before Thomas tried to ask her for a phone number. Anita aimed for the big Tube sign in the distance. *Who had invented these horrible shoes?* Kicking the heels off, she ran the rest of the way barefoot, shoes in her hands.

She burst into the station, hunting for the toilets. The smell of vomit and urine punched her as she entered the room. She quickly put her shoes back on, wishing she had wellies instead. Her stomach turned upside down as she gingerly stepped over a puddle of something unidentifiable. Gritting her teeth, she shut the cubicle door behind her.

Anita slumped on the toilet, letting her tears run; tears of relief that she had survived the ordeal, tears of disgust over the experience. But she knew she had to get up; she knew she had to get home. Washing her hands and face, she rushed to the platform. She didn't care that her mascara had started to run. She didn't care about anything. All she wanted was to be back home.

As the Tube sped towards Paddington, Anita watched her reflection in the window. Her mind feeling blank and numb, she had no idea how to deal with what had just happened. The experience was still too raw.

Once on the train home, she sank deep into the seat.

> I'm on the train home. Thank you for playing along

> Thank goodness. I'll come by tomorrow to hear everything. Message me when you get home

Anita burrowed her body into the seat, willing the world to disappear and her mind to stop hurting. The lights of London sped past her window, but Anita's eyes filled with bitter tears and she didn't see any.

CHAPTER 3

Anita woke up with the usual niggles and a heavy feeling in her lower abdomen announcing her period.

"Shit, shit, shit!" she swore as she curled up into a tight ball, sobbing. The whole effort ended in failure. She lay on the bed, defeated, her heart shredded to pieces. Her sobs turned into strangled cries while she tried to regain her composure again.

Ok, ok. I need to calm down. Just calm down. Breathe, ... ok, breathe. I need to stop stressing. It's not the end of the world. I knew it wouldn't work the first time I tried. I knew the chances were slim. Yes, I had hoped that it would, but nothing's lost yet. I will try again. I have to. And I will succeed. I've done it once; I can do it again. There's nothing else to do. ... There, that's better.

Anita took another deep breath in and let it slowly out before getting out of the bed. She dragged her feet to the bathroom to sanitise her menstrual cup. She normally didn't mind having a period. Using a cup made it pretty easy. However, for a woman trying to get pregnant, and going into so much trouble for it, the knowledge that it didn't work had the power to shatter her will.

Three weeks later, Anita alighted the London bound train again. All dolled up, she chose a different part of the city for her 'get pregnant' escapades. Nothing would be worse than running into Thomas again.

The night began in a similar fashion to the first one. She entered a busy night club with loud music playing. Lots of suitable objects milled around, but nobody gave her a second look. Maybe Thomas was an exception and Anita had misjudged most men? Why did nobody want to sleep with her? She didn't get it. She was wearing a seductive dress and smiled at everyone in a way she hoped said what she was up to. Still, she had to talk to several men before finding a keen subject. After almost giving up, he sidled to her with a playful smirk on his face.

Sex in a bathroom cubicle had its advantages, the biggest one not having to undress. Anita didn't have to endure his skin on hers. This man just pulled her skirt up and entered her. He obviously only wanted sex; and didn't even try to kiss her once. It suited Anita fine. She didn't need to fake anything; he was eager to just please himself and move on. No escape plan needed. He lost all interest in her afterwards, and two hours later, Anita was on the train back home. While she still hated the experience and knew that he had used her as much as she had used him, she found it easier than last month.

But two weeks later, her period came again. How long would she be able to go on like this? She wanted a baby, but these outings drained her soul as much as they sucked all the energy from her body. But she had to go on. She had to. What else could she do?

So, the next ovulation time, Anita jumped back on the train to London, hoping for another quick affair. Choosing a different club again, she scanned her surroundings.

"Stella, it's so nice to see you here," a voice boomed behind her.

Oh bugger, Anita's heart sank. Out of all the places in London, he had to be in the same one as her. What a horrible coincidence. She turned with a pretend smile to face Thomas.

"I hope your sister was ok last time."

"Yes, she was fine. How are you?" Anita tried to conceal her disappointment. His presence marked the end of the quickie in the bathroom.

Why the hell is he in the same club? That's so unfair. What should I do? I don't owe him anything, and I definitely don't want to have sex with him again, either. That's clear. He's too nice, and I actually enjoyed talking to him last time. The sex just spoiled it all and now I can't even look at him. No, I don't want to be here with him. I can't go through the physical ordeal with him again. I just can't, once was too much. I'll have to leave and find a different club. There's nothing else to do.

"Can I get you a drink?"

"Yes, can I have a glass of wine, please?" she said. "I'll meet you at the bar in a second."

Ducking to the ladies, Anita exhaled. She had to act fast. Making sure Thomas had walked off towards the bar, she sneaked out of the bathroom, heading for the exit. A pang of remorse filled her body at leaving him there, but it had to be done. She didn't like running away like this, but it had to be done. Twice in a row might mean something to him, and she couldn't risk that. She bolted outside and down the road, almost colliding with two young women.

"I'm so sorry, girls."

"You are in a hurry, aren't you?" they giggled giddily. "Running away from someone?"

"I am actually," Anita responded. "My ex."

"Oh, come with us. We'll help you escape!" they laughed again.

Anita followed them to another club. It didn't take long for a couple of men to join their little group. One took a particular liking to Anita, and she didn't stop him. This club had a little courtyard at the back and so they retreated in there soon after under the pretence of looking for a quiet place to talk. They both knew what would happen, and it happened fast. At least for him, Anita never reached orgasm. But she had never expected to; she would have to actually enjoy the experience. After the act, the man disappeared inside. She didn't even know his name.

Anita left the club straight away, feeling like such a whore. She had sex with three different men in the last three months. Anita had never imagined that would happen to her, never in her wildest dreams. Third time lucky, she repeated her mantra and rubbed her lower abdomen, willing the sperms to reach her egg.

CHAPTER 4

"I'm pregnant," yelled Anita, dancing around the bathroom with the pregnancy test firmly grasped in her hand.

"Yay, hun, congratulations. How amazing! You must be absolutely stoked," said Zara when Anita called her with the good news.

Anita beamed. What a perfect word for it. Zara's dad was from New Zealand, and so frequently she used words not spoken in England much.

"Yes, I am stoked," she laughed, unable to conceal how excited she was. From now on, her life was going to be perfect. And even when two weeks later Anita's morning sickness started, it couldn't dampen her high spirits. The doctor had confirmed her pregnancy a week earlier, and she had her twelve-week scan booked already. Obviously, the counting began from the moment of fertilisation, so Anita was already one month in.

Anita was flying on a happy cloud. She had planned to enjoy the pregnancy; she had planned to read all the books and articles she could find and follow all the rules and advice given. What she had never expected was for her nausea to become as bad as it had. No matter how many times Anita told herself it would pass soon, the constant vomiting and dizzy feeling put a damper on the experience. And her mood soon reflected her physical state. The sense of hopelessness just lingered on; the sense that the sick feeling would never end and that her suffering would stay until birth. It took all her strength and will to push through.

"Let's see your baby," said Zara when they walked into the radiology clinic two months later.

Anita squeezed her hand, seeking some encouragement.

"Anita Wright? Room number one," the sonographer said after they had waited for a while.

"Please, lie down on the table, lower your skirt and underwear and pull your top up a little."

When Anita did that, the sonographer put a cold gel on her stomach and picked up the scanning machine. She moved it all over Anita's exposed area, watching the screen in front of her. Anita stared at the screen below the ceiling, not really understanding what she was looking for and what she should be seeing.

Finally, the sonographer said, "I cannot find the foetus."

Anita's heart skipped a beat, the room suddenly spinning around her. "What do you mean you cannot find the foetus? I am pregnant, aren't I?"

"Technically, you are pregnant, but I can't see the heartbeat; it's not showing on the sonograph. I would like to do a vaginal examination, if you don't mind."

"Of course," Anita peeped, grasping Zara's hand.

"Please, go to the bathroom first. Afterwards, if you could please take your underwear off, lie back down on the table and cover yourself with this blanket. I'll be back in a minute."

Anita got up as if in a dream. She walked to the bathroom, tears streaming down her cheeks.

The baby is not there. There is no heartbeat. How come? Where is it? It must be there. Why wouldn't it be there? How would that happen? ... No, the sonographer must be wrong and she'll find it now. She must. The baby is there. Of course, it is. It has to be.

Lying on the bed again, Anita watched the sonographer taking out a long probe.

"I will insert this into your vagina. Just relax, it won't hurt. You can watch what it sees on the screen."

Anita stared at the screen, tears pushing their way out, blurring her vision.

"I have found the egg. Unfortunately, it is not developing. The yolk sac has calcified and stopped providing nutrients to it. I'm very sorry, but your pregnancy is not viable."

Zara held Anita's hand. Anita squeezed it so hard her ankles turned white.

"I'm sorry," the sonographer said again. "I will send a report to your doctor, who will discuss the next course of action with you. You can get dressed now."

Anita dressed in a daze; her mind clouded. She left the examination room without a word, followed by Zara. They hugged outside, both crying.

"I'm so sorry, Anita. I'm so sorry."

"In my opinion, the best will be to let nature do its job."

Anita stared at the floor in the doctor's practice, only half listening to what he was telling her. She felt so numb from the emptiness that had filled her, the sense of dread overcoming her entire being.

"There's a surgical option as well, but it causes more stress to the body. The choice is yours. What would you prefer?"

"Ms Wright?"

Anita raised her head, her expression blank. "I'm sorry. What did you say?"

"I asked if you would rather leave it to nature or have a surgery to remove the egg."

"I think I'll let my body deal with it. It should know what to do."

But does it, really? Does it actually know what to do? Why didn't it recognise that the egg is not growing? Why didn't it expel it earlier? Why did it wait until 12 weeks and made me sick for nothing? I'm so furious with my body, so angry with it right now. It made me so sick for so long for nothing, for absolutely nothing. It betrayed me completely and let me suffer. ... Or maybe it didn't. Maybe it didn't stand a chance. Maybe it was my head that caused all this and kept the egg in. I so want this baby and so maybe my body didn't dare to get in my way. But now I know this pregnancy is not happening, my body can do what it needs to do. I will have to trust it.

And her body did. Two days later.

Anita curled up on the bed, her stomach burning with unbelievable cramps. Something was happening, and Anita had no way of controlling it. A sudden weird feeling made her move faster than she had ever moved before. She barely made it to the toilet before a huge blood clot left her body. She detected more movement as another one made its way out. Undressing fast, she jumped into the shower just seconds before another clot dropped. It splattered on the shower floor, droplets of blood spraying the glass. The bleeding grew heavy, with clots literally rolling around the tray like balloons. Anita hunched in the shower, crying and quivering, frantically trying to wash the blood down the drain. She had lost so much blood that the area looked like a murder scene.

Where is all this blood coming from? How can there be so much of it? This can't be right. What if I bleed out? I need help.

Anita opened the shower door, noticing a few droplets of blood dripping off the glass onto the shower mat. She searched through the pile of clothes on the floor for her phone.

"Zara, thank goodness," Anita said after Zara finally picked up. "I'm having a miscarriage, but I think I'm losing too much blood! Can you come, like now? Can you take me to the hospital?"

Anita waited in the shower, sitting in a heap in the corner and letting the water run down her spine, soothing her stressed body. She washed the blood of herself as well as possible, but she had no way of stopping the stream of blood and clots still coming out of her.

"Anita, where are you?" she heard Zara calling as she burst into the house.

"Up in the shower!" she shouted.

A rapid sound of footsteps pounded on the stairs and Zara flew into the bathroom.

"Are you ok? How are you feeling?" she gasped, breathless.

"Quite weak, to be honest. And tired. What shall we do? I can't stop the bleeding. Maybe I should stuff a towel between my legs; otherwise, I'll bleed all over the car."

Zara grinned a victorious grin and pulled out adult diapers from her bag. "These are Grandpa's," she said. "Grandma said to take them."

Zara lived with her grandparents, taking care of her grandfather, who had Alzheimer's.

"Hopefully they work. I'm bleeding lots," said Anita, turning the water off and pulling the diaper on.

In the meantime, Zara brought a loose dress from her room. "This will be better than trousers."

Anita nodded. She dried her body and put the dress on. As she stood up she had to lean against the wall; her head was spinning too much. Zara had to support her down the stairs and into the car.

Sitting Anita in the passenger seat, Zara jumped into the car, speeding off. The hospital was about 20 minutes away; they had no time to waste. While Anita sat in the car, the bleeding had settled, but her stomach was still cramping.

"We're here. Can you walk or shall I get the wheelchair?"

"I think I'll manage."

Anita got up and the moment she did so, a huge clot released.

"I need the loo. Really fast."

Zara rushed her inside, pushing her into the bathroom, which was straight by the entrance.

"I'll tell them you're here," she shouted after shutting Anita in the cubicle.

Anita pulled the incontinence pants off and rolled the blood ball into the toilet.

How the hell am I going to clean this?

She scrunched up her nose at the sight of blood all over the seat and her inner thighs. She sighed and grabbed some toilet paper, wiping the blood off her legs first. As much as she didn't want to, the bloodied pants had to go back on. With more toilet paper, she cleaned the seat from the worst and flushed it all. Anita stood there, watching the bloody mess going down the drain before unlocking the door and walking to the basin. Wetting a wad of paper towels, she walked back to the bowl, cleaning and drying the toilet seat as well as she could. Scrutinising her work, she frowned. It wouldn't do. She would have to do it again.

Zara rushed in. "Come, they're waiting for you."

"The toilet seat needs a better clean. I've tried, but it's still dirty. I need to do it again."

"Don't worry about it, Anita. You need to take care of yourself now. I'll tell them about it, don't worry. Come, they'll see you now. I have filled in the paperwork already; you only need to sign it."

Anita let Zara hurry her into the reception area where a nurse was already waiting with a wheelchair. She gave Anita a sheet of paper. Anita didn't even read it, just simply adding her signature to the bottom. She was sure that Zara would have filled it correctly.

"You will have to wait here while Ms Wright goes to the doctor," the nurse told Zara.

Anita tried to protest. She wanted Zara with her. She needed Zara to be by her side. But with her body and mind weak from the loss of blood and the entire ordeal, she only waved while the nurse wheeled her away.

CHAPTER 5

"This is going to be uncomfortable."

Anita lay on the examination table, her legs up in stirrups, her mind running in circles.

"We need to open you up more to examine what is still inside. Are you ready?"

Anita closed her eyes. "Yes, I'm ready. Do whatever you need to do," she said, resigned to her fate.

The doctor inserted a device into Anita's vagina. It probed and pushed on the sides of her opening, stretching her in ways she would have never thought possible. A nurse assisting the doctor said something, but Anita didn't catch what it was. Not that she wanted to know. They were both peering inside her, pulling bits and pieces out.

"Do you mind if I invite another doctor for a second opinion? I suspect something is still inside, but I can't reach it."

Anita muttered, "That's ok."

She had lost all her dignity already.

Two more doctors came, discussing her intimate parts. Well, not her intimate parts, but the situation happening behind them.

Invite the whole hospital, if you must. I don't care who sees what anymore, thought Anita.

Finally, the doctor said, "I believe we got everything out. Do you want to keep it?"

Anita's surprise must have mirrored in her face.

"Some people bury their unborn foetuses," the doctor said in explanation, reading her expression correctly.

"This wasn't a foetus, though. Was it?" Anita whispered. "It was a calcified egg."

"No, you're correct," the doctor agreed.

"I don't want to keep it. Thank you for the offer, but you can dispose of it here."

"Very well. You need to rest now; the nurse will take you to your room. You'll need to stay here for a few more hours still for observation. Part of your developing placenta was attached to the uterus. It sometimes happens, so we had to scrape it out."

The nurse wheeled Anita into a private room where Zara already sat waiting for her.

"Oh, Anita. Thank goodness. How are you doing?" she asked with concern.

"I'm doing. The whole hospital came to check out my spread legs."

The nurse smiled apologetically. "It had to be done. The doctor couldn't get some of the tissue out."

"I know, she told me. But it was still quite the experience."

"Can I get you anything? I'll bring you some food, a cup of tea, and water. You need to gain more strength, but is there anything else you need?" asked the nurse, while attaching a drip to Anita's arm to get more fluids in.

"No, I'll be ok. Actually, could I have some painkillers? I've got quite the headache."

"Certainly. I'll bring you some. The drip will help as well. You've lost a lot of blood and your body is reacting the only way it knows, with pain. You'll start feeling better soon."

The nurse left the room.

"How are you really doing, Anita?" Zara moved next to her bed, holding her hand. "And I don't want to hear fine, because I'm sure you are not fine."

How am I doing? I'm sad, disappointed, angry, hopeless and sore. I'm embarrassed, defeated, and tired.

"I just need to sleep now, Zara. I'll be fine. Thank you for being here," she smiled at Zara and closed her eyes.

But Anita wasn't fine. Her soul was healing slowly and her body even slower. After spotting almost every day for six weeks, she got her first post-miscarriage period. And it came with a vengeance. Anita bled heavily with the cramps' intensity curling her toes. Painkillers made no difference; she even had to take time off work to get through the first two days. Then, the cramps stopped and the bleeding slowed down and settled, but didn't stop. The bleeding just didn't stop. Anita bled for the next 25 days, only to start again after a brief five-day release. The bleeding grew lighter, but the pain during the first few days and the length pattern stayed the same. Like before, she had a few bleed-free days in between before her third period arrived.

Anita shrieked in despair. *When will it stop? When will this finally stop?*

At least she had the cup. How would she have coped with a pad or a tampon she didn't know. That would make it unbearable.

"I'll have to go to the doctor," she told Zara the next day.

"I'm bleeding again; it's the third month of bleeding. That can't be normal, can it? I think that something is definitely off."

"Yes, have it checked out, even if just for your own peace of mind. Your body is obviously fighting something."

"You might be right. I'll wait for my period to stop, if it does, that is," Anita rolled her eyes, "and book an appointment."

Anita sat at the doctor's practice after her period had finished two days prior. He had examined her but found nothing out of the ordinary.

"It is possible that your body forgot what it is supposed to do. A miscarriage has a big impact on the entire system and it can take a while for the body to deal with it. I will prescribe you a strong medication, steroids actually; they should help. Take one a day in the evening with food and try to avoid doing any physical activity afterwards. I'm hoping the medication will kick your body back into action and it will remember what it is supposed to do. If these don't help, we'll look into something else. There are a few other avenues that we could explore."

The pharmacist gave her a long spiel about the medication, stressing the 'take it with food and don't exercise' parts. It sounded like a killer drug and with only five huge pills in the packet looked like one too. Anita hesitated to take the first one; the side effects written on the enclosed leaflet sounded horrendous. She held the pill between her fingers, examining it from all sides.

You little, odd, horrendous pill. What are you going to do to me, I wonder? Are you going to help me or kill me? Who knows. Oh well, it has to be done. In you go.

Anita sighed, gingerly laying the pill at the back of her

tongue. She swallowed it and went to sleep. The next morning, she started to bleed again.

Maybe that's what the pill is supposed to do, Anita grumbled. *I don't know what this body is doing anymore. Maybe it's just like the doctor said and it forgot completely what it's supposed to do.*

In the evening, Anita popped a second pill in, and an hour later, things started to happen. Not knowing what pregnancy contractions felt like, Anita guessed that they couldn't have been much worse than her pain. Curled up in a little ball on the bed, whimpering like a newborn puppy, Anita wished for the pain to go away. Her stomach hurt all over and now and then, a sharp stabbing pain shot through it. The pain blinded her sense of reality and time. Anita did not know how long she lay in one spot, unable to move, unable to get up and call for help. Time had no impact on her. She could only clutch her stomach and wait, and hope that it would soon be over.

A strong cramp twisted her body and a hot, fiery burn froze her. Another huge contraction followed and, as quickly as the cramps had come on, they all stopped, leaving only a twinge of pain in their wake. Stretching her legs as long as possible, Anita relieved her limbs, sore from the position she had been in for so long. Willing her body to move, she rolled onto her side and sat up.

Well, this was something. What actually was it?

Anita shook her head, trying to clear her mind. She made her way to the loo, barely keeping her cup in. It felt heavy and needed emptying. She pulled it out to discover not only blood, but also a piece of something else.

What the hell is this?

It resembled a piece of meat! Baffled, Anita stared at the contents of the cup. She leaned towards the vanity drawers, searching for some kind of container. Rummaging through, she grabbed an old pill bottle, popped the piece in it and closed the lid. *The doctor might want to see it. I'll call the practice tomorrow.*

As she had planned, Anita called the doctor's practice the first thing in the morning. After explaining to the doctor's receptionist what had happened, they advised her to bring the piece in for testing. She dropped it off straight away and two days later the doctor called her with the results.

"The lab said it was a placenta tissue. It must have still been attached to the side of your uterus and the steroids loosened it. It would have caused all the bleeding issues you have had because your body didn't know what was happening. You don't need to finish taking the pills, if you feel well. I believe you will be ok now."

"I had already stopped. I had taken only two and when the tissue came out, I stopped. I've been feeling better. I'm still bleeding, but it is painless and very light now. I feel more like myself again."

"Perfect. Come back if anything changes."

Anita put the phone down. Her body could now finally start its healing process. The almost constant pain she had felt the last few months had stopped, but her heart and soul still hurt. She still longed to have a baby, and this episode didn't deter her from trying to achieve her dream in any way. If anything, it made her want it even more. She was so close.

CHAPTER 6

"I'm going to London tonight," Anita told Zara on Saturday morning.

"You can't be serious!" Zara exclaimed.

"Why not? It's been four months. I'm well again. My period has settled back into its normal routine, and I'm ovulating. It's the perfect time."

"The time might be perfect, but I was hoping you were done."

"Because of a miscarriage?" Anita raised her eyebrows high. "I won't stop just because I had a miscarriage, Zara. So many women have miscarriages and they still keep on trying. Did you know that every third woman experiences a miscarriage at least once in her life? It is actually pretty common, it's just not talked about."

Anita did a lot of reading on the topic during her healing period. Knowing that she wasn't the only one had helped her to come to terms with the ordeal.

"I knew you haven't given up on having a baby, but I was hoping you gave up on the one-night stand idea," Zara whispered.

"Zara, I know you are worried. And I don't enjoy doing it either, far from it, you know that." Anita shrugged, a shiver running up her spine. "But I really, really want to have a baby. Please, understand. I'll message you again every half an hour. I promise."

The dusk had set in when Anita arrived in London. She stayed close to Paddington, scouting a good club. On Saturday night, the city buzzed with groups of merry people. She followed the sound of music to a brightly lit venue with a queue of people waiting to get in. *With a queue, it must be good,* she reasoned.

Paying the cover, she tagged to a bunch of girls in front of her. In her mind, it made her look less desperate. They walked down a long corridor which ended on a balcony with two long staircases on its sides. These wound down alongside the walls, leading to an enormous dance hall below. Anita leaned against the balustrade, surveying the area. The bar filled the entire back wall, with rows and rows of various bottles on mirror shelves. A huge spinning disco ball hung from the ceiling, shooting little discs of light at the swaying crowd. The music coursed through Anita's body as her face spread in a huge grin. What a place; what a wonderful place. The amazing atmosphere deafened her hesitation. If Anita didn't have a very important job to do, she would have liked to dance the night away there. But not that night.

The cocktail menu looked as amazing as the venue. Anita hadn't heard of many of the drinks on offer before. How would she ever choose? At the end, she ordered a Tequila based cocktail called Cacti Punch. She might as well have something special while searching. Sipping her drink and playing with the little paper umbrella, she scanned the crowd in front of her. Her heart sank with disappointment. Couples and groups of women crowded the bar and the dance floor; the space absent of any single men.

Tonight will be a fiasco, a complete disaster, noted Anita after walking around the hall several times. *Maybe I should dance the night away like I had wanted to instead. Yes, that's what I'll do and try again next month. But first, I need a fresh drink.*

A young, dark-haired man approached her on the way to the bar.

"Can I get you a top up?"

Anita beamed at him. "Sure, thanks."

"What are you having?"

"Cacti Punch."

"Sounds interesting. I'll join you; I've never had that before. I'm Martin, by the way."

"Stella."

Anita kept her fake London name. After meeting Thomas twice already, she didn't want to compromise her identity.

Martin bought their drinks.

"Where's your group?"

"I'm here alone. I wanted to go out, but none of my friends did."

"What a shame. Such a pretty girl and here on her own? That's not good, that's not good at all."

Anita flashed him a smile, but his remark made her uncomfortable. She couldn't quite put her finger on it, but he acted odd, in a sleazy sort of way. But with no other single man around, Anita didn't have much choice, so she decided to give him a go.

"So, where's your group? Don't tell me that you're here alone, too."

"Oh, they are here and there," Martin said, waving his arm around. "Just a few boys, nobody that important. You wouldn't want to meet them, anyway. They're a rowdy bunch. You know, typical young Brits."

This small talk was killing her, especially because she didn't find him at all amusing or appealing. Anita needed to speed things up to get this business done and dusted, so she threw him a bait.

"I'm going out for some fresh air. It's pretty stuffy here. I'll see you later. Thanks for the drink."

"Hold on, I'll come with you; fresh air will do me good."

The fish had taken the bait.

"It's busy here tonight," said Anita as they walked out onto the street.

"It's always like this on the weekends. Do you want to find a quieter place?"

"Yes, why not."

Anita dreaded this moment, but she also wanted it to be over already and go home where she could nurse her bruised soul and cry herself to sleep.

"Don't worry, I know just the spot."

Martin led her around the corner into a little courtyard with a bench and a single tree. Anita aimed for the bench, wanting to sit down. But Martin had different plans. He grabbed her violently, pushing her onto the bench, and bending her over the back of it. Pulling her dress up and her underwear down in one swift motion, he entered her with violence. Anita had no time to react. She tried to fight him off, but he held her down hard. All she could do was to gasp in pain.

"Isn't this what you wanted, slut? It's what you've been asking for, isn't it?"

He thrashed his body into hers while Anita sobbed.

"Oh, shut up, you whore. I'm giving you only what you wanted. Nothing else."

With a man much stronger than her, Anita struggled to free her body. The world had disappeared, only the pain stayed. The pain and the shock. How was this happening to her? With one last powerful and rough thrust, he finished. Crying, Anita pulled her underwear back on, but when she straightened up, he smashed her across the face. Anita hit the ground, yelping in pain. A trickle of blood ran down her forehead, her entire body numb. In a quick step, he towered above her, planting a brutal kick in her side.

"Is this what you sluts like? Is it? It is, isn't it? I've given you only what you asked for, so why are you wailing? Just stop that stupid noise already or I'll hit you even harder."

Anita curled up into a ball, protecting her soft body parts, while he continued beating her.

"Hey! What are you doing?! Leave her alone!"

The kicking stopped, and Anita heard steps running away.

Then a young woman's voice spoke to her, "Are you ok? Can you stand up?"

Anita turned her head in a daze, squinting to focus on the pretty face framed in blond hair looking at her with concern. "My angel," she mumbled, before closing her eyes again.

"No, don't sleep. You can't sleep now. Wake up. You have to get up." With the woman's help, Anita got up and crumbled onto the bench.

"You're bleeding," the woman said, pulling out a packet of tissues. She dabbed one on Anita's cut, cleaning her face.

"I couldn't catch him; he must have slipped into one of the side streets. Are you ok?" said a breathless young man, dropping down on the bench beside them.

"She's pretty banged up," the woman told him.

"Can you walk?" she asked Anita. "There's a 24/7 clinic nearby."

Anita nodded, and the young couple lifted her up, each

supporting her on one side. Anita hung in between them, her handbag dangling in front of her like a pendulum counting up her steps. She stumbled painfully, every step hurting more than the one before. Sharp pain shot through her ribs whenever she moved and her pelvis area felt like on fire. Even though they walked only for about five minutes, to Anita it seemed like eternity. At last, the bright clinic sign flashed ahead.

The young people pulled her inside the waiting area, rushing to the nurse. "This woman got attacked. She really needs help."

The nurse looked Anita over. "This cut will need stitches. You'll have to wait for the doctor. Sit down and I'll bring you a numbing cream and a bandage to put on it for now and do a quick vital signs check."

The nurse brought over a First Aid kit. She bandaged Anita's head and asked her a few questions about the attack.

"Please, follow my finger." Anita followed her finger as well as she could and then blinked several times when the nurse shone a torch into her eyes.

"You don't seem to have a concussion. Good. I'll bring you a form to fill in."

"How long will she have to wait for the doctor?" the young woman asked.

The nurse scanned the waiting room. "I'll prioritise her because she's bleeding, but it will still be at least 30 minutes. We're quite busy tonight."

She turned towards Anita. "Can you wait that long?"

"Yes, I'm sure I can," Anita murmured.

"I'm sorry, but we won't be able to wait here with you," the couple apologised.

"I understand. Thank you very much. I think you saved my life," Anita whispered, squeezing both of their hands. "Thank you so much. You don't know how grateful I am. I wish I could give you something in return."

"Don't mention it. Everyone would do the same in that situation."

"No, not everyone. Many people would just ignore it and walk away. You are special. Thank you."

Anita gave their hands one last squeeze and let them go. As she watched them leaving the waiting area, tears welled in her eyes. She was left alone with her pain.

Her phone beeped. Zara! She had forgotten to message her. Barely concentrating on the screen, she wrote,

> I'm ok. Can't talk now. Will message soon

Anita put the phone back into her bag and tried to concentrate on the clinic form.

How could I have been so stupid? I should have listened to Zara; Zara knew what could happen. She warned me, but I was so stubborn and thought I knew better. Well, this will teach me, won't it?

After returning the form back to the nurse, Anita ducked into the loo. She pulled off her knickers, shaking with disgust. They were stained with both blood and semen, creating a revolting mix. Scrubbing them vigorously, she stuck them underneath the hand drier, keeping her eye on the door in case someone walked in. Anita looked at her reflection in the mirror, her eyes grew wide and she gasped. An enormous bruise coloured her left cheek and her lip had a deep gash with dry blood stuck in it. Her heart skipped a beat at the sight of the large bandage across her forehead. Tears filled her eyes, tears of disappointment and frustration. She could have been killed! If it wasn't for the lovely couple, she would have been killed!

The door creaked. Anita scrunched the knickers in her palm and fled into a cubicle. She dropped onto the toilet, tears forcing their way out again. *How could I have been so stupid? So horribly stupid?*

The outside door shut again as the woman had left. Anita peeped out, making sure the room was actually empty. Stepping back to the hand dryer, she continued drying her knickers.

"The doctor will see you now, Ms Wright," said the nurse after Anita had returned to the waiting room.

"Thank you," said Anita, following the nurse to the doctor's room.

"Good evening, I'm Doctor Beth. How are you?"

"Pretty sore," said Anita truthfully.

"Can you tell me what happened?"

Anita recollected her ordeal as well as she could remember, while the doctor typed a few notes into her computer.

"I'm sorry you got attacked. Let me look at your head. But first, take these for pain; I'm sure you have quite the headache."

"Ok," the doctor continued after Anita swallowed the pills. "We will sew the wound now. Please, lie down on the examination bed."

Anita lied down, hissing in pain, and closed her eyes. She found it easier to deal with the world without seeing it.

"The local anaesthetics the nurse put on the wound should already be working, but it will still hurt a little."

The doctor cleaned her forehead with wet gauze, leaving it on her wound. Anita found the cool material soothing as she listened to the doctor getting everything ready.

"I'm going to start now."

The doctor pulled and pricked Anita's skin, but it didn't hurt as much as her back.

When the doctor had finished, she said, "I'll send a report to your regular doctor. They will make an appointment to remove the stitches, but if you bleed from the wound or you have oozing discharge, go there straight away. Ok?"

Anita nodded.

"Now, we'll check your body. Can you please take your dress off and stay standing up?"

Anita did as she was told, wincing when pulling the dress over her head. Every little move sent jolts of pain to all parts of her body; jolts so strong that they shot through her like lightning, burning their way in.

The doctor checked her back first. She pushed here and there and prodded her soft areas without talking.

"Please, lie on the bed again, on your front this time."

Anita obliged, summoning all her will to do so, while the doctor continued the examination.

"Can you turn on your back, please? I know it hurts, but I have to check you thoroughly."

Accompanied by loud grunts, Anita managed. The doctor pushed on Anita's stomach, searching for painful spots. She found none.

"You were fortunate, very fortunate, actually. You have nothing broken or burst, only lots of bruising on your back. It will be sore for quite a while; I will not lie to you. Have you got enough painkillers at home or do you want a prescription?"

"I reckon I've got enough," Anita said.

"Good. Go home now, take two more pills and from tomorrow take them whenever needed, up to the recommended dosage on the packet. Go to your doctor immediately with any new pain or if your symptoms worsen."

Anita turned to leave.

"And one more thing," the doctor stopped her. "As this was an assault, it will get automatically reported to the police. They will call you and you can choose to lodge an official report to start the investigation."

"Oh, I see. I will expect their call then. Thank you very much."

Anita paid for the treatment at the reception, thanked the nurse, and limped outside. She stood in front of the clinic for a while, wondering where the train station was. Not recognising anything around, she returned to the clinic.

"Excuse me, which way to the Paddington station?" she asked the nurse.

"The station is about 10 minutes away, but there is a Tube station just around the corner. Go right, then turn right at the first crossing and you will see it."

"Thank you."

Anita found the station easily and, once on the train, messaged Zara.

> On my way home now

> Thank goodness! I'll come to see you tomorrow

"Anita, what happened?" exclaimed Zara upon seeing Anita's face.

Anita almost jumped into her friend's embrace, melting into it, tears streaming down her face in an endless waterfall. "I've been so stupid, Zara. So stupid. You were right all along," she blurted. "It was so dangerous. Just stupid. I should have listened to you. Why didn't I listen to you?" Anita's body shook with violent sobs.

Zara held Anita tight, allowing her to talk things out before asking, "What happened last night?"

Anita's body tensed. "I got attacked, ... and basically raped."

"You what?"

Anita recalled the whole evening while Zara stared in shock, taking in every word.

"You know what the worst part was? When he was kicking me and calling me a whore, I knew I deserved it. Deep down in my soul and in my stomach, it felt right. I've behaved like a whore. I've had sex with more men in the last half a year than in my entire life before. Men I didn't know. This felt like a justified punishment."

"You definitely didn't deserve this," said Zara. "And don't let any horrid man make you believe you did. Remember why you did it. You want a baby. And yes, it was dangerous, and it was stupid. But nobody has the right to treat you like this. Nobody."

"Thank you, Zara. I have learnt my lesson. I'm done with this. I'm done being stupid. I'm never ever having sex with another man in my life. I'm never ever going to put myself through such danger."

"We will work this out, hun. I'm sure we will. You will have your dream baby, you will."

Anita glanced at Zara gratefully. "I so wish you were right, but at this moment, I don't see how. I don't want to give up on my dream but ..."

"Something will happen that will change things, you'll see."

"I'm so happy to have you in my life, Zara. I don't know what I would do without you."

"Oh, you would be fine. But I'm happy to have you in my life too and to be in yours, of course. Even though you've been extremely problematic lately, young lady."

Anita chuckled, "I'm sorry, Miss. I'll try to be better from now on."

"I should hope so," said Zara in a stern voice before continuing in her normal one. "Have the police called you yet?"

"No, and I don't want to talk to them. What am I going

to say? - Oh yes, officers, I got attacked and raped after going out with a guy, wanting to have sex. That won't flow well with them, will it? No, I'll rather tell them I didn't see his face, so no point in reporting it because they won't be able to catch him, anyway."

"I don't know, Anita. I suppose you should report it. He can't get away with this. How many women has he done this to already and will still do it to? You know his name, at least, and you know how he looked. Your testimony might be the last piece of puzzle the police needs to actually apprehend him. Please, don't be embarrassed. They don't need to know why you did it. All they need to know is that you liked the guy and went for a walk; he pulled you into the courtyard and attacked you. You've got nothing to be ashamed of. You are the victim here."

Zara was right, of course she was, but Anita was ashamed. She wanted to hide away from the entire world and forget about everything. She hated herself for what she had put her body and soul through; and she never wanted to do it again.

"You're right, Zara. As always," Anita sniffed. "Ok, when the police call, I will report it."

"Thank you. I'm sure it will do you good, too. You will be able to put it behind you and get on with your life."

With what life? A life without a baby is not a life. I know I will always be unhappy; deep down inside me, I will always miss something. My life will always have a hole that I cannot fill.

Tears streamed down Anita's face again, and she couldn't stop them.

"Oh, Anita, it will be ok, I promise."

Anita said nothing, but while sobbing wished to have the strength to believe Zara. She wanted to believe her, but couldn't. Things would never be ok. Never.

CHAPTER 7

This can't be true. Please, don't let this be true. I can't believe this. Not now. Not like this!

Anita stared at the pregnancy test in her hand in despair. The lines showed a clear, positive result. There was no doubt about it. As much as she wanted to get pregnant, she didn't want to be pregnant with the man who attacked her. She had tried so hard to forget about the entire experience, which, given the fact her body still hurt like hell, she had bruises turning all colours across her back, and a slowly healing wound on her forehead, proved to be quite impossible. But she could never forget if she had a child to remind her of it all. And she would never forgive herself for bringing a baby born from trauma into the world. A baby born from pain. No, this wasn't fair, this wasn't fair at all.

Anita collapsed on the bed in a sobbing heap. She couldn't remember a day when she didn't cry. She cried so much in the last few months that it surprised her to have any tears left to shed. Her life had turned into a tragic story and it was she who had caused it. Her and the stupid idea of getting pregnant with men she didn't know. What an idiot she was; what a complete idiot.

When the police called at her a few days earlier, Anita told them what happened to her. She described Martin and the entire situation, omitting the fact she did this to get pregnant. She didn't tell them how often she had done the same previously, either. Recalling the experience to them cost Anita a lot of strength, but they were understanding and didn't question her virtue at all. They only wanted the facts, nothing else. However, they did tell her that the chances of them finding Martin were pretty slim. Anita didn't mind at all. She never ever wanted to see that man again. She never wanted to look into his eyes and see the hatred she felt while he was kicking her. Which, if they arrested him, she might have to. She would have to testify against him then, and how would she do that? How would she stay calm, especially now, when she was carrying his baby? How would she do that? What's worse, how will she ever be able to look at her child and not see her attacker? How? Goodness, what a mess she got herself into!

Later that day, Anita called Zara. She had to give her mind time to process what had happened and pull herself together.

"Zara," Anita hesitated after Zara picked up the phone, "I'm pregnant."

"What wonderful news, Anita," Zara exclaimed, pausing as the reality sunk in. "Wait! You are pregnant after the attack? Oh!"

"Yes, exactly. Oh."

"How are you feeling about it, hun?"

"I'm not sure. I've been finding it hard to forget and now I will have a child to always remind me of it. I'm not sure what to do."

"You'll keep the baby. It's simple," Zara stated. "You've been through too much not to."

"Yes, of course I will. Not keeping the baby didn't even cross my mind," said Anita. "Although, I expect I'll need help to come to terms with it. I might need to visit a therapist or a healer of some sorts."

"Great idea. You will get through this. You are strong, stronger than you think. And I'll help you. You can always rely on me, Anita. Don't forget that."

"Thank you, Zara. I'll go to the doctor tomorrow to confirm and follow on from there."

The urine test at the doctor's practice only confirmed what Anita already knew. She was definitely pregnant.

"How are you doing, Ms Wright? Are you still sore after the attack?" the doctor asked while inspecting the bruising and her wound.

"Yes, it still hurts, but it is healing. My body will be fine soon."

Anita stopped talking, unsure how to continue. "Um, I wanted to discuss something with you."

"Yes? What is it?"

"Well, I am pregnant after the attack and, to be honest, I don't know how to deal with it. How am I going to cope with the fact that this baby is my attacker's baby? How can I live with myself and this child? I can't even imagine what my life will look like. I've wanted a baby for so long, but not like this. I don't think I can do this." Anita's eyes welled up.

"It will not be easy, you are right, but there are avenues we can explore. I can refer you to a psychologist who will help you. I know several brilliant specialists who you can talk to. They will help you analyse the situation and give you strategies to work things out; strategies to cope with your grief and regret. With such help, I'm sure you will manage. Is this something you would be interested in trying?"

"Definitely, that's what I actually wanted to do. I'm willing to try anything at this point. I've been so stressed and anxious and everything I do upsets me."

"You've been through a lot. Give it time. Time is the best healer. How were you coping with the attack before you learnt of your pregnancy?"

"I was getting there. It was hard to forget with the pain, but I was doing fine, considering. I journal and it helps me greatly to put all my feelings and thoughts on paper. I actually thought that I was doing well, processing the event in my own way, until the positive test sent me back to the beginning. No, it sent me deeper than I was before."

Anita folded her hands in her lap, looking at the floor so the doctor didn't see her tears making their way out.

"That's good to hear. Do you want to approach a psychologist straight away or would you rather wait until the first scan before you embark on this journey? Given your previous miscarriage, there is a slight chance this pregnancy won't be viable either. What would you like to do?"

Anita looked up with teary eyes. "I think I'll wait until after the scan. If the egg is not developing, I might not need a psychologist at all."

"It might still be good to talk to someone about the attack, though. I'll write you a referral now and you can always use it if you feel like you need it. Personally, I would recommend you approaching someone."

Anita nodded. The doctor printed out a few forms and handed them to her, a lab form for a blood test, a radiology request form, and the referral.

"I would like you to have the scan at week eight already. I think it will be better than waiting until week twelve."

"Thank you, I agree. The sooner I know, the better."

"You are almost five weeks now, so call the radiology

centre to book an appointment today. They tend to get quite busy."

"I will. Thank you."

"You're welcome. We're finished for today, but call the practice anytime you need to see me again."

Anita thanked him one more time and called the radiology clinic the moment she walked outside. She managed to get the booking she needed. Having the appointment scheduled had given her a certain sense of action. She had something to prepare for, but what would she see on the screen? What news would she learn? What news was she actually hoping for? She didn't know.

"I'm sorry, Ms Wright. I can't detect a heartbeat, but let me check one more time."

"No, I can't hear any heartbeat at the moment. However, this doesn't mean that the foetus is not there. The embryo might be just too young. You might have fallen pregnant a week or two later than you had calculated. I would like you to come again in two weeks' time for a re-scan, and then we'll know for sure."

Anita just nodded, too numb to even talk. She made another appointment for the required date and left the clinic, wondering what to think and how to feel. Zara had other commitments, so she couldn't ask her opinion. She had to figure this out on her own.

Well, the day of conception is correct. I am already eight weeks pregnant. I couldn't have fallen pregnant at any other time. I know that the sperm can stay alive for a few days, but that still wouldn't make much of a difference. The heartbeat should have already been visible, that's clear. So, there is no baby. This is good news, isn't it? Yes, this is actually great news. I don't want this baby. Rather than living with a constant reminder of the attack, I will stay childless. As much as it hurts me and tears me apart, it is not worth the stress and anxiety. Yes, this is good news, indeed.

An enormous boulder lifted off her shoulders. Anita straightened up her back and raised her chin high. All of a sudden, the world turned brighter; the sun shone, and the birds sang just for her. Oh, what a lovely day this is turning to be. *Now, I only have to wait two weeks to have this confirmed and go through the miscarriage process again.*

A dark cloud passed in front of Anita's sun. She frowned at the thought of the miscarriage.

Well, it has to be done.

At the next appointment, the sonographer confirmed the embryo wasn't developing. Another natural miscarriage was out of question, Anita just couldn't go through the blood loss and emotional rollercoaster again, so she had asked the doctor for surgical removal. The doctor agreed and arranged a date for her hospital stay, only two days later. She had no time to even get her mind ready for it.

Anita sat in the waiting room at the hospital, picking on her nails and cuticles. Zara couldn't stay with her there, but promised to pick her up afterwards. Anita had to go under general anaesthetics, and so wasn't allowed to drive by herself that day.

"Ms Wright?" the nurse came to get her. "Come this way, please."

Anita followed her into a small room.

"You can change into the hospital gown here. Please, place all your belongings into this bag."

Once alone, Anita folded her clothes into the bag and slumped on the bed, her thoughts flitting around her brain, not making much sense. The feeling of hopelessness had overtaken her mind, forcing anxiety to attack her body. As much as she wanted to stay calm, she just couldn't.

The nurse came back. "Please, swallow this medication and I'll take you to the theatre shortly."

Anita just managed to send Zara a quick message before the nurse arrived again.

"I will take you in with the bed, so please lie down."

How odd to be wheeled around the hospital in a horizontal position, thought Anita.

The bed shook a bit every time the nurse opened the doors with it and the walls sped past rapidly, without Anita being able to find her bearings. All she could do was watch the lights on the ceiling above her. This surreal experience didn't help her nervous mind at all.

"I'm doctor McKay, I'll be your surgeon today," a middle-aged doctor awaiting her in the theatre said when they had arrived. "Don't worry, this is an easy surgery and it will be over soon. Are you ready?"

Anita gave a feeble nod of agreement.

The anaesthetist approached her, putting a mask on her face.

"Inhale deeply, you will soon fall asleep. One, two, three, four ..."

Anita opened her eyes and tensed, trying to remember where she was. It took her a while to recognise the little room the nurse had ushered her into upon her arrival to the hospital. She breathed a sigh of relief. It was done.

"Oh good, you're awake. How are you feeling?" the nurse said, walking into her room.

"I'm ok," Anita whispered, her voice sounding hoarse.

"Here, have some water."

The nurse passed her a glass. "Are you hungry? Do you want to eat?"

"Yes, please." Anita's stomach rumbled; she didn't realise how hungry she was until the nurse had asked.

The nurse brought a tray with sandwiches, juice, and a small bowl of ice-cream. Anita devoured all of it in mere seconds.

The door opened with Zara flying in. "Are you ok? How are you feeling? Was the surgery ok?"

"I'm good, Zara, don't worry," Anita smiled at her best friend. "But if, by some miracle, I ever get pregnant again and it is not viable, I'm having the surgery. I am never again going through a natural miscarriage if I can help it. This was so much easier. They put you to sleep, take it out, and then even give you some ice-cream afterwards."

"I'm glad to hear that."

Anita's mind flashed back to her first miscarriage. The tremendous loss of blood and the horrible ball-like clots scared her. She saw them in her dreams for weeks afterwards; they were the worst. The surgery, on the other hand, was a breeze. No pain and no blood. Easy.

"Let's wait for the nurse and find out when I can go home. I'm ready to face the life again," said Anita with a newfound vigour.

Let the healing process begin.

CHAPTER 8

"I can't believe you're getting married next month!" exclaimed Anita, dancing around Zara, who was trying her wedding dress on. "The dress is amazing. You look absolutely beautiful."

Zara twirled in front of the lounge mirror, dressed in a white lacy dress. Anita picked up the thin tiara decorated with delicate purple flowers, which had arrived from the dressmaker, and inserted it into Zara's blond hair.

"Stunning, just stunning. Chris's jaw will drop all the way to the ground when he sees you."

"Are you sure it fits me well in the back? It feels a bit tight. Maybe I've put some weight on since the last fitting," said Zara, stretching her arms forward to test the size.

"It looks great. Hold on, I'll bring the bedroom mirror to show you."

Anita ran off, coming back with a long mirror. She stood it up so that Zara could see her reflection. "See? It's perfect."

Zara inspected her back. "I guess so. It still feels a bit tight, though. Oh well, it's just for one day anyway, so it will have to do. Now try your one on," she said, pointing at a smaller box on the table.

Anita opened it. Inside was a light purple dress with thin straps, decorated with the same flowers adorning Zara's tiara. She rushed off to the bathroom to get changed. It fit her perfectly. The dressmaker did an excellent job.

"You look amazing. We both look amazing," clapped Zara in delight.

The previous year had been hard, but Anita's life had been slowly returning to normal. Helping Zara with the wedding plans had helped Anita to forget about her plight. The only physical reminder being a barely visible scar above her left eye. A bit of a concealer and nobody would ever know what she had been through. Nobody, but Anita herself.

The soul healing was taking longer and, on some nights, Anita still woke up in sweat and fright. However, this had been happening less and less often and the last month, only once. Anita had a few sessions with a therapist; at first, she tried to manage on her own but quickly realised she couldn't. And the sittings proved priceless in helping her to shake off the idea that she deserved to be hurt for her behaviour. She recollected exactly what had happened to the therapist and why. The therapist had offered practical strategies and procedures to deal with the blame and personal guilt, and now Anita's body and mind were almost whole again.

Almost. She still longed for a baby. More than ever. Going to the shops proved difficult as she teared up whenever she saw a pregnant woman or an infant. At this moment, however, Zara's happiness took over her own wants. Zara had always given her so much and had helped her through all the bad times. So, now it was time for Anita to return the kindness. Afterwards, she could plan her own happiness.

"Anita! Yoo hoo, Anita, are you there?" Zara waved her arms in front of Anita, who was staring out of the window lost in thoughts, trying to get her attention. "Are you ok? You blanked out for a while."

Anita smiled. "Sorry, I've got too much on my mind, I suppose. Yes, I'm good. What's in the last little box?"

Anita nudged Zara.

Zara opened the smallest box. A white handkerchief, embellished with the little purple flowers that were on both the tiara and Anita's maid of honour dress, laid neatly folded in it.

"This must be for Chris's suit pocket. It's so pretty. I love how all the clothes are matchy-matchy."

Anita hugged her friend. "It's going to be a beautiful wedding. Chris is so lucky to have you. And I am too," she added, squashing the brief pang of jealousy towards Chris.

Anita liked Chris. He and Zara were meant for each other. However, the couple didn't keep it a secret that they wanted to try for a baby soon after the wedding, and that troubled Anita. Not that she didn't wish them to be happy, but how could she continue being friends with Zara, if she burst into tears every time she saw her pregnant and later on with a child? How could she possibly do that?

"Anita, you've gone again," Zara touched Anita's arm. "Let's pack this up and go over the things needing to be finished. I have little time left. 26 days to be exact. Oh my, I'm going to be a married woman in 26 days. Let me introduce you to Mrs Zara Howard. How funny it sounds!" Zara giggled.

"It sounds perfect. It suits you. You know what I don't like? Let me introduce you to Mr and Mrs Chris Howard," said Anita, scrunching up her nose. "This always grinds me. As if a woman is just a part of a man."

"It's not that bad, Anita. I don't mind it at all."

"Well, you keep it then, but I'm really glad it won't ever happen to me. I'll stay Ms Wright until my very last day here on earth," Anita snapped.

Zara gave her a funny look.

"I'm sorry, Zara. I didn't mean it in a bad way."

"I know, and you're forgiven. Just sometimes, your words come out of your mouth before your mind has had a chance to think them through," Zara added.

"I know, and those words are usually not nice. Just you wait when I'm old, they will be absolutely horrible," Anita sniggered. "Nobody will want to be around me then."

Anita surveyed the wedding venue; the big day had arrived. The small garden restaurant, decorated in white and purple, looked perfect. Bouquets of white daisies and purple lilies sat on each table and in tall vases around the area. White and purple streamers hung from the wooden beams above, complementing the white and purple tableware and details. Further at the back, a wedding arch dominated the garden, covered in daisies with a few purple lilies adding a splash of colour. Several rows of chairs stood arranged in front of it, almost all already occupied with the wedding guests. Under the arch, the registrar waited with a nervous-looking Chris Howard. Anita watched him from the window in the little room where Zara was finishing her preparations.

"Chris is nervous," she giggled. Zara rushed to the window.

"Good! My whole body is shaking."

"Don't worry, the wedding will be perfect. You've done such a great job organising it and the place looks amazing. Are you ready? All your guests are here now," said Anita, watching the last people arriving.

"Yes. Where's my dad? And is Mum ready, too?" Zara asked anxiously.

Her mum and dad had arrived from New Zealand a few days before the wedding day, and were still very much jet lagged. Especially her dad, who suffered from bad motion sickness, was still recovering.

"Yes, your mum is sitting in the front row beside your grandparents. Let me see where your dad is."

Anita peeked outside the door, spotting Zara's dad waiting behind them, rubbing his hands together.

"And your dad is ready too, looking as nervous as Chris."

"Oh no, we all are. I hope it all goes well. Let's get this thing over and done with, then."

"Yes, let's do it. Give me one minute. I'll do my duty," said Anita, rushing out of the room.

"She's ready," she told Zara's dad on her way to the little three-piece string orchestra to tell them to start playing. Squeezing Chris's arm in support, she took her own spot beside the wedding arch.

The music began to play and Zara, on her dad's arm, walked out into the garden. All the guests turned to look at the beautiful bride. Chris melted at the spot, his nervous expression turning into a huge smile as his gaze followed his future wife walking down the aisle. The two of them locked eyes. Anita beamed, filled with complete happiness for the special couple.

After the vows, the yeses, and all the signatures, Anita hugged the newlyweds. "I love you guys so much. Have the most amazing life together and thanks for all the support you have given me. I couldn't have wished for better friends. Now, let's get this party started, shall we?"

Zara hugged Anita back. "Thank you for helping me with the wedding. I love you, hun."

"And I love you. Have the best of nights."

"We will, we surely will."

The blue afternoon sky soon turned into a starry night. The wedding guests danced and talked, ate and drank, and Anita joined in all the festivities. She couldn't remember the last time she felt this good.

When the newlywed couple had retired, to the loud cheers of everyone present, Anita stayed on to help to tidy up the venue. She rubbed her heavy eyes, struggling to keep them open.

What a night; what a special, beautiful night.

Warm happiness spread throughout her body. Zara deserved only the best, and this was her happily ever after. Now to get her own.

CHAPTER 9

How interesting, thought Anita while searching the internet.

It'd been almost a year since Anita's attack. 11 months and 17 days, to be exact, not that she was counting.

Anita scrolled further down the page. Her search term 'artificial insemination' had returned a few interesting results. She skimmed past the agencies, or clinics as they called themselves, she had contacted previously. *Nah, waste of time.*

However, a clinic claiming to be helping single women caught her eye. "Are you a single woman longing for a baby? Come and talk to our team. We will find a solution for you," Anita read aloud.

The ad certainly sounded hopeful, and if she was at the beginning of her journey, she would have contacted them. However, after all the rejections, Anita held a deep grudge towards these clinics.

Maybe I could give this one a call, she mused.

Wait, what's this? Home insemination? Anita clicked on the link. An agency in the States was offering to send women sperm to attempt their DIY artificial insemination at home.

Anita read, "We send either fresh or frozen sperm, and detailed instructions ... you can choose your donor from our extensive database ... health and safety screening of all donors makes this option safe and viable ... your privacy is guaranteed."

Anita's heart beat faster. She had never heard of this option, but she would be keen to try it. Her shoulders slumped as she read the next sentence. "At this moment, we don't deliver to international locations."

"Damn!"

Of course, they don't. And it looks like that even in the States, only people residing in some states can order from them because each state has a distinct set of rules. How odd. So, people living in the United States don't have equal rights regarding this? What if someone lives close to the border of the state, which allows insemination at home, but they are in one not allowing it? Could they order the kit to a friend's house in the other state and still do it? That would work, wouldn't it? Anita shook her head in despair. *I don't know why I'm even wondering about this. I don't have any friends in the States, anyway. Bugger.*

Anita typed the search term 'home insemination UK' into the bar. She scrolled through the results but found nothing similar available to British women. She pored over the blogs and articles about home insemination instead. If she found a donor herself, it would be worth a try. Apparently, the process was relatively straightforward. A donor ejaculates into a clean cup. A woman takes a syringe, one of those needless ones, and injects the sperm into her vagina, aiming for the cervix. The other option was using a menstrual cup, with the donor ejaculating into the cup and the woman inserting the cup in and leaving it in for a maximum of 12 hours.

Anita wrinkled her nose. *So, I would insert the cup in and the wrigglers would swim up? Hmm, I'm not so sure. Wouldn't they just stay sitting in the cup? Maybe standing on one's head would help them out. How fun would that be?* Anita giggled.

She breathed a sigh of relief, her mind clear after such a long time of darkness. Finally, she was doing something towards her dream again. For so many months, just thinking about it hurt, images of the attack flashing through her mind. The therapy and Zara's wedding had helped and as a result Anita gained a new will to live. And this home insemination method had given her new hope and determination; it energised her whole being.

Now she needed to locate a suitable donor.

Hmm, how do I find one of those? How will I actually know a man is suitable? Neither of my male friends would do. Hell, I wouldn't want any of them to be my baby's biological father; they wouldn't do at all. And I just can't ask a random man on the street, can I? Good afternoon, sir. I'm searching for a sperm donor. Are you available? Anita chuckled. *And how would I know the donor is healthy? I have to make sure the donor doesn't suffer from any hereditary or contagious diseases. He would have to get tested for sexual diseases as well; I wouldn't want to catch anything. God, how stupid was I? I went out with men I didn't know, men who probably changed partners often, maybe every night, never worrying about this. My want to have a child blinded my judgement completely. I would have happily brought that child into this world. Honestly, I was such an idiot.* Anita shook her head in dismay.

One blog also warned about the legalities of the process. Finding your own donor meant the person knew he was the biological father and became a legal guardian. They advised to engage a lawyer to draft an agreement with the biological father stating that he is giving up all his rights to legal guardianship.

Yes, such a brilliant piece of advice. Nothing would be worse than a donor coming back after a few years and claiming rights to my child. No, a signed agreement would have to be done.

Anita typed 'dating agencies' into the search bar. *Wow, so many of them,* she thought, scrolling through the pages and pages of results. *There are more results here than for artificial insemination.*

Anita opened a few of the UK based ones. With most, she would have to register before being able to search, which she didn't want to do, but a few allowed her to search through the men without it. She looked at some profiles, not really finding anyone suitable. Some were good-looking men, but their profiles clearly conveyed the message they were seeking either fun and games or a serious relationship. Obviously, nobody on these sites wanted to donate their sperm. *No, dating agencies would be another waste of time.*

Zara, I need you, sighed Anita.

She had to talk this through with someone, and Zara was that someone. Unfortunately, she wouldn't be back for another two weeks. She and Chris went to Hawaii for their honeymoon before flying to New Zealand to spend some time with Zara's dad. Her mum stayed in England to help with Zara's grandfather while she was away. Zara kept on sending Anita photos. Hawaii was stunning, such beautiful beaches and all the flowers; it was definitely a place Anita would love to visit one day. The two newlyweds were having the time of their life so Anita would have to wait; bothering Zara on the honeymoon with her issues would not be fair.

Anita turned the computer off, sighing again.

I'll just have to wait for Zara's return. I'm sure she will have some ideas. Zara always knows what to do.

"So, what's the thing you need to pick my brains about?" said Zara, sitting in Anita's kitchen, sipping a cup of liquorice tea.

Anita smiled at her best friend. Zara had been back from her honeymoon for almost two weeks before Anita brought the topic up. She wanted to give her enough time to settle back into a normal life after a month away.

"Well, I suppose you know I didn't give up on my dream of having a baby."

"Yes, I knew you didn't. I just didn't want to talk about it until you did."

"I might have come across a solution while you were away. A viable solution. One I would be perfectly ok with physically and emotionally."

"Go on," said Zara, perking up in her chair.

"I did some more internet research while you were away. Things have changed in the last year, or maybe I wasn't putting the correct search words in before, which is more likely. Actually, that's what it would be. I had never thought to search for that before." Anita rolled her eyes. "But I discovered it is possible to do an artificial insemination at home."

She studied Zara's face for a reaction.

"Tell me more. How does it work?"

Anita told Zara what she had learnt online; all about the sperm transfer, health checks, and involving the lawyer.

"That's the easy part. The hard part is getting the right man. I've looked at some dating websites but found nobody suitable. Where and how do I find the donor, Zara? That's where I'm lost."

Zara thought it over, biting her bottom lip. "It sounds like a great idea. And with all the health checks and no physical contact, it would be so much safer for you and easier than what you had gone through. We should have done more research last year. We were both so stupid to let you go to London."

"I know. What were we thinking? Well ..., rather, what was I thinking? You were against it from the beginning, but went along with my idea because I'm so stubborn. I was such an idiot. I wish I had listened to you," Anita said, shaking her head in disbelief. "I could have died that night. If the young couple were not there, it could have ended up very differently."

"It could have, but didn't. You are safe and well."

Zara bit her lip again. "Now, how do we track down your perfect man? We could try an ad in the newspapers."

Anita's eyes almost popped out.

"Don't look so alarmed," laughed Zara.

"And what do you suggest we put in it? A single woman searching for a sperm donor?"

"Exactly. I would write something like: A single woman searching for a sperm donor for artificial insemination. Conditions: clean police vet, willing to undertake a health check, willing to give up child's legal guardianship. And your phone number. That should do it."

Anita considered her friend's plan. "I don't know. Do you reckon it's a good idea to splatter my name and phone number all over the world?"

Zara laughed, "It won't be all over the world, silly. Only here in Maidenhead, and maybe Reading or Windsor. It's probably not worth putting it into big national newspapers. It would just become one of many ads there and you might get more pranksters calling you. And we wouldn't write your name there either."

"Pranksters. What a nice name for the idiots. And they will call; you bet your marriage on it. They will. I don't know, Zara. A lot of people will call just for fun."

Anita thought about the idea again, "And I didn't want

anyone here in Maidenhead, or in the nearby areas, so nobody would find out who the father is."

"I know Anita, but for practical reasons, a person from here would be better. You don't want to travel somewhere up to Scotland, do you? And you never know, Mr Right might be living in the next street. I would try it if I were you. What have you got to lose? None of the people who know you will ever find out you advertised for a donor. I can't see anyone checking the phone number on the ad in case they know the person advertising," said Zara. "Well, you could also always get a new cheap phone and a SIM card to keep your own phone number safe, you know?"

"Ok, I'll do it," Anita agreed after a moment of silence. "I'll get a new phone, and you'll come with me to all the meetings with these pranksters."

"I'll be happy to. I won't let you go alone to meet a stranger ever again."

The ad got published on Monday, and by Wednesday, Anita had had enough. She had expected lots of prank calls, but she had never imagined to what extent. Her phone kept on ringing and beeping basically nonstop at all hours of the day and night. People called her by many names, with a whore, a slut, and a bitch definitely the favourite, but many called her a cow, as well as by other animal names. She received lots of religious messages, citing parts of the Bible she was apparently breaching. One person left her a voicemail ordering her to stop this campaign or the hand of God would smite her.

Some of them Anita laughed off. For some reason, even though she wasn't a religious person, she found the religious messages harder to ignore.

Lots of men just offered her sex. They were not very

imaginative either. The favourite message being, 'Pick me, I'll give it to you good.' *How pathetic.*

Several messages only said, 'Call me, I'm interested'. However, neither of them turned out to be serious. After she had explained what she needed, one person said, 'Wouldn't it be more fun to just have sex?' While another suggested, 'Yes, that sounds good. So, are you going to do a striptease for me while I'm getting done?' And yet another, 'I'm all for it, but I'll need help. Is hand job an option?'

Anita didn't have time to waste with these morons, these 'pranksters', as Zara had called them. Zara answered some calls when she was with Anita. She found most of them funny. To her, they were not personal, and she just brushed them off. But in Anita's case, they dug deep, piercing the very spot where her longing for a child sat.

"Just forget about them," said Zara, while shaking her head. "None of these people would tell you the same straight into your face. They're just keyboard warriors. They know their identity is hidden, so they write and say whatever they want to. I'm sorry, Anita. You were right. This wasn't the best idea I've ever had. Actually, it might have been one of my worst."

"No worries, Zara. You couldn't have known. Hopefully, the calls stop soon."

But the phone calls and messages kept on coming. Anita had to turn the phone off at night to get a break and leave it at home whenever she went out. At least they didn't use her real number.

What a brilliant study to human psychology this experiment would make. Give people a bait and watch them take it. How could so many people attack an unknown person with such vengeance? 'Love thy neighbour' for sure. The religious messages and calls were the worst of the lot. While Anita wasn't a churchgoer, she believed in an entity of some sort; but given the horrible mess in the world, the entity couldn't have been the caring, all mighty ikon people worshipped. Anita more believed in nature and in her own inner power and strength, and the support of her closest, rather than in someone else guiding her journey on earth.

After two more weeks, Anita dreaded the phone ringing. The constant buzzing annoyed her too much. And even though the calls and messages had eased off in the last few days, those that came through didn't grow any mellower. Anita groaned as the phone rang again, picking up the wretched thing.

"I've got a sex offer for you," a deep voice said on the other side the moment she said hello.

Without a word, Anita turned the phone off.

"Another sex offer," she said to Zara, who was sitting opposite to her at the kitchen table.

"I'm sorry, Anita. This was a stupid idea. I didn't realise how low humans can go. I knew you would get stupid calls and messages, but this? It's like every single man in the borough has called you."

"I don't think it was only men. Well, yes, only men called, but quite a few messages sounded as if a woman wrote them. I must have insulted many righteous women on the block. ... Crikey, how grateful I am we didn't put my name on the ad. Can you imagine? It's not like my name is Jane. Not many women are called Anita."

"True. That was lucky."

"I'm ready to throw this SIM card away, to be honest."

"Yes, you might have to. I hope this experiment didn't hurt you. I'm sorry I came up with such a stupid idea. I obviously didn't think it through."

"Zara, you couldn't have known how bad it would get. Don't worry, the messages and calls are not doing me any lasting harm. It's true that some of them hurt and some of them hit quite deep, but mainly they're just annoying. Once the card is gone, I'll be fine."

Zara scratched her head. "I'm glad. But you could always just keep the phone turned off. You don't have to throw the card away."

"Nah, I don't think so. If I just turn it off, I'll want to check it again soon. You know, in case someone normal has contacted me. And then I'll have to read the same messages all over again. It'll be better to get rid of it completely. I'll give it two more days and if nothing happens by Tuesday night, in the bin the card goes."

As Anita said, she did. On Wednesday morning, she opened the bin, cut the SIM card in half and threw it in with relish. *Off you go, stupid people,* she thought. *Call as much as you like now. I don't have the stomach for you anymore. What a journey this has been! So many attempts and so much failure. How exhausting.*

CHAPTER 10

"I've got a man for you," Zara cried, bursting into Anita's house.

"What do you mean? Where? And who?" Anita enquired, with hope rising inside her.

"Well ..., rather Chris has, I should have said. I shouldn't be taking credit for something I have nothing to do with, should I?"

"I see, so Chris is playing a matchmaker now, is he?" said Anita, raising her eyebrows.

"No, no, it was purely accidental. I told him about the text messages and phone calls, and he said we could have expected it. You did, I didn't. I assumed people were better, I guess. But they're not. Most people are garbage, given the chance." Zara shook her head.

"So, tell me about the man your matchmaking husband has discovered."

"Can I get a cup of tea to go with it?"

"Yes, I'll make you some tea. Just spill it already."

Anita pretended to get angry at her friend.

Zara laughed, "I'm spilling it, don't worry. So, Chris's got a new colleague. Like he's not new new, but he started just before we went on our honeymoon and then Chris was away for so long, so he doesn't know him too well yet. But from what he had heard, and from the few brief conversations he's had with him, he figured this man is your perfect fit."

"Okay," said Anita slowly. "What does he teach? Or is he an admin?"

Chris was a teacher, teaching English at several local colleges.

"He teaches Spanish. Apparently, he's just arrived back from Spain after spending about 15 years there. He came back home after his failed relationship. I don't know all the details, but it sounds like he wanted a child and his partner didn't. So, George, did I mention his name was George?"

Anita shook her head.

"I didn't think so. So, George had ended the relationship and came back home. Well, not home. He doesn't come originally from here, which is another plus, because apart from his colleagues, nobody really knows him in Maidenhead."

"Ok, this still doesn't make him the perfect fit for me, does it?"

"Oh yes, it does! Let me finish," Zara said. "He doesn't want another relationship; he just wants a child. And ... he's a gay." Zara beamed at Anita in triumph. "He would be on board with artificial insemination. In fact, I'm positive that he wouldn't have it any other way," giggled Zara meaningfully.

Anita studied Zara's expectant face. He sounded plausible, but .... Yes, a big but clouded her mind. A huge and significant but. "But if he wants a child, he's not likely to give up legal guardianship, is he? He will want the child to know he's the father."

"Yeah, you would have to talk it through. You are pretty set on this condition, huh?"

"I am. You may think I'm being bossy or overpowering, but I don't want to discuss every single thing with the biological father only because they did sooo much work by kindly donating the sperm. This will be my baby, living in my house, growing up with me. I don't want to consult someone all the time. The donor could butt in whenever he felt like it and tell me I can't do things the way I want to do them. He could tell me I can't put the child into a particular school or teach him or her at home, if I wanted to do that. Or that I can't take the child for a trip overseas or even move there if I ever wanted to."

"Oh, yes, you're right. I didn't consider any of these. Hmm," said Zara, "well, we'll meet with this guy and see what he has to say. See if he's up for it and if he agrees to your conditions."

"Wait! Has Chris already spoken to him about me? Or have you?" Anita jumped up in alarm.

"No, no, we haven't. Chris told me about him a week ago and yesterday, he spoke to him properly to get to know him better."

"Oh, good. It sounded like he had already told him." Anita sat back down.

"So ..., what do you think, Anita? Is it worth a shot? He sounds like the best and safest option we've come across so far. You can't lose anything by talking to him, and I will come with you, of course."

Anita pursed her lips, considering it. He ticked most of the boxes. His school would have already police vetted him to teach children, he wouldn't want to have sex, and he would likely be willing to undergo a health check. Even though the legal guardianship could be an issue, Zara was right. He sounded like the best option she had had. She would likely always regret not meeting up with him.

"Ok, set up a meeting."

"Yay. I'll get onto it straight away." Zara ran around the table and hugged her friend. "Let's all go for dinner; Chris can join us, too."

"No, that sounds too much like a double date. Can we rather go somewhere informal? Just for a cup of tea, you know? I wouldn't want to scare him away."

"You got it." Zara squeezed Anita again.

A well-dressed man with short black hair and dark-rimmed glasses walked into the café. Anita and Zara snapped to attention; their eyes locking.

That must be him, Anita thought, suddenly feeling very nervous.

The place was quiet at 1.30 in the afternoon; right in between lunch and afternoon tea time. They chose this time specifically.

The man surveyed the room and aimed straight for their table. Zara and Anita rose in welcome.

"Mrs Howard, I presume," he said in a friendly voice, his eyes darting from one woman to another.

Zara stepped forward with her outstretched hand. "Zara, please. And this is Anita."

"George Pearce. Nice to meet you, ladies."

"Please, sit down." Zara pointed at an empty chair on the opposite side of the table.

Once they were all seated and the waiter had left with their order, George asked with his eyebrows raised, "Now, please tell me what this meeting is about."

"I gather my husband didn't tell you much?" Zara asked.

"No, he said his wife," George motioned towards Zara, "had a friend," he looked at Anita, "who's got a certain proposition for me. I'm all ears."

"Anita, do you want to explain?" Zara nudged Anita.

Anita's throat tightened, and the words stuck in her throat. Her fingers fidgeted with the hem of her skirt under the table as she struggled to start. Her heart pounded in her chest and red colour rose up to her cheeks. It was ok to talk about her dream with Zara, but now, she was supposed to share it with a complete stranger. Despite him looking open minded, this was proving difficult. Zara's and George's eyes burned into her, both of them waiting for her explanation. Anita steadied her voice and mumbled.

"I want to have a baby."

"Anita, you will have to speak up," said Zara.

"I want to have a baby," said Anita in a louder voice. "However, I, um, don't like physical contact. I do like men; I just don't like sexual contact. Which, as you imagine, prevents me from getting pregnant."

She bit her lip, not sure what to say next. *Why is this so difficult?* She had practiced the speech at home, but it all got mixed up now, half of it gone out of her head. With hesitation, she continued.

"I contacted several agencies last year, and they all declined my application. Apparently, I'm not a suitable candidate. The only reason I have come up with is because I don't have a partner and they just can't be bothered to cater to single women. I have tried stupid things," Anita swallowed hard, "things that almost cost me life, but nothing has worked so far." Anita grasped her cup of tea for comfort. Now, she had to ask the big question.

"Are you ok?" Zara asked. "Do you want me to continue?"

Anita glanced at her friend. "No, I will do it. But thank you."

Staring into her cup, Anita said, "Since then I have learned that it is possible to do artificial insemination at home. However, I'm missing a donor. Some agencies in the

States, well, I found one, can send sperm to women, but they don't ship internationally. And I didn't find anything similar here in the UK. I have even put up an ad searching for a donor."

"Oh, I saw it," George jumped in. "That was you?"

Anita whimpered, "I gather the whole of England saw the ad, judging by the number of messages I got. Most of the messages and calls were mean and nasty, with lots of religious people condemning my actions and a huge number of men wanting to have sex."

Zara chimed in. "Blame me for the idea. I didn't expect such a response. Never in my dreams. Honestly, how can people be so horrible?"

"People say more than they would into your face when hidden behind their phones, some maybe not even intending to cause pain," said George.

"Yes, I assume many of them wouldn't have realised how hurtful their messages were," said Anita.

"So, where do I fit into this?"

I'm sure you know already where I'm going with this. You must, thought Anita. *But I guess you want to hear it from me.*

"Well ..., I'm sorry if this is encroaching on your privacy, but Chris told us you wanted a child and your partner in Spain didn't. So, you broke up and came back."

"Yes, true. I don't mind Chris telling you."

Anita plucked up her courage and said, "So, I was wondering, would you be interested in being my sperm donor?"

George leaned back in the chair; his composure rigid. "What exactly would it mean for me?"

"It would mean that you would have a child who you could visit, take out for trips and fun outings, but the child would legally be mine. We would have to sign an agreement specifying the conditions. The thing is, I would want you, if you accept, to give up your legal guardianship rights." Anita fixed George in a stare.

"So, I would be a father without being a father."

"Umm, yes."

"When do you need to know my answer? I want to think this through."

"Is one week enough? I'll be ovulating in about two and a half weeks, if you don't mind this personal information, so if you agreed, we could already try then. I don't expect it working the first time, but the sooner we start, the sooner I could get pregnant."

George thought for a bit. "One week should be enough. Do you want to meet here in a week's time again?"

"Yes, perfect. Thank you so much for considering it."

"Well, it is an interesting proposition. I just need to sleep on it a few times."

After George had left, Anita hugged Zara. "He sounds interested. Fingers crossed, he agrees. Oh, I won't be able to sleep the whole week," she laughed.

"I'll be holding all of my fingers crossed for you." Zara hugged her back. "Shall we go home now? I can't wait to tell Chris."

CHAPTER 11

Anita tapped her foot on the floor, waiting for George at the café. The last week had dragged, each minute lasting hours and hours lasting days. Her heart raced with anticipation as she awaited the news that could change her life forever. Her mind filled with hope and dread.

What if George says no?

The more she thought about him, the more she knew he was the perfect donor. He was the one she wanted to have a child with. Or was she so desperate? Her patience almost gone, Anita picked her nails, trying to hush her noisy mind.

Zara's absence made things both better and worse. Anita would have loved to have someone to talk to, but she thought that not having Zara with them might make her and George more comfortable discussing the issue. Well, George really. She shared everything with Zara, anyway.

The door opened and Anita perked up. A young couple walked in and sat at a table by the window. Anita didn't like waiting, but she had arrived early. George still had another five minutes left. She normally drank herbal or fruit teas, but in her anxious state had ordered a cup of strong Earl Grey.

Get a grip on yourself, Anita. You don't have to be such a wreck. If this doesn't work out, another door will open. You got this. He's not your only option. She tried giving herself a pep talk. It didn't work. She needed to know his answer already, one way or another.

Exactly on time, George walked in. He waved to Anita and, maybe noticing she already had a cup, stopped at the counter to order his drink before heading to her table. They shook hands and sat down. George didn't look calmer than Anita, his eyes avoiding hers. After the initial pleasantries and the almost compulsory weather talk, they both fell quiet. The waiter had come and gone with George's tea, but they still avoided the topic. Anita knew she should pop the question, but a lump in her throat prevented her from speaking. *Oh, come on, ask him already. You can't sit here like this the whole day.*

"Um ..., so what do you think? Have you had time to think about the idea?"

"I have," George answered. "It wasn't a straightforward decision to make. I'm sure you know that." He looked up at her before shifting his stare back into his cup.

"Naturally. I understand."

Please, tell me already. Tell me now!

George obviously needed to gather his courage as well.

At last, he straightened up and said, "I have decided to be your donor."

Anita's whole being exploded in happiness. A tremendous weight lifted off her shoulders. She barely stopped herself from hugging him.

Her face beaming, she burst out, "Thank you, thank you so much. That is amazing."

The world turned a brighter colour all of a sudden and

Anita's thoughts danced in great excitement, already imagining the baby she would have.

"I do have some conditions, though," said George.

"Yes, yes, of course, and so do I, as you know already. We can write all the conditions down and engage a lawyer to draft a proper agreement," sang Anita, adding, "I'm happy to pay the lawyer's fees in full, of course."

"Sounds good. Do you want to do it now and here, or shall we go somewhere quieter?"

The café started filling up for afternoon tea. A private place sounded better. But where? Anita didn't want to take him home, not yet. Where else could they talk in private?

"The library's got meeting rooms. We could ask to use one," Anita suggested.

"Let's try."

They finished their drinks, stood up and, after paying their bills, left the café. The mild weather of the late spring welcomed them outside, the sun matching Anita's mood, happy and bright.

The librarian told them their meeting rooms were all full, but she could offer them a relatively private desk in the corner. They sat down at the table and Anita got her notepad and a pen ready, handing a sheet of paper to George.

"Maybe the best will be if we both write our conditions on a piece of paper first."

"Yes, sounds good to me. I have a few notes written already," he said, pulling a folded sheet of paper out.

"Oh, good. I'll write mine then."

Anita bent over her paper, writing the three points that mattered to her: health check, legal guardianship, and visiting rights. She didn't need anything else. She wanted the donor's sperm to be healthy and to have full legal control over the baby's upbringing. The visiting rights were just for George's benefit. She glanced at George.

"Are you ready?" Anita asked.

"Yes. This is all I want to include. I don't need to add anything else at the moment."

"Ok. My first point is a health check."

"The same here," replied George.

Anita raised her eyebrows.

"Yes, I would like you to have a check-up too, to make sure there's nothing we should know about. If I am to become your donor, I want to know that you are healthy and that the baby won't be affected in any way."

"Fair enough; I can do one. Hopefully, we can both get an appointment pretty soon. I've got only about 10 days left until I ovulate again and I want to try this month already. Well, if we can't, I guess it will have to wait, but I've wanted this for so long already that it is hard for me to do that," Anita said in apology.

"No need to explain. I'm happy to try as soon as we are both ready."

Anita smiled.

"My next point is legal guardianship. As I said before, I would like you to give up all your legal rights to the child."

"My next point as well, and I will give you the full legal guardianship, but only under these conditions," said George, passing her his piece of paper.

Anita read them aloud,

"1. Visiting rights

- visits at times agreed on by both, but at least twice a month

- day long trips at times agreed on by both, but at least twice a year

- yearly holidays at times agreed on by both, but at least once a year (once the child is older, from approximately six years of age)

- invitations to child's birthday parties and special occasions (like school plays, graduations and other celebrations)

2. Legal guardianship

- Anita will write a will in which, if something happens to her, the full legal guardianship passes to me

- Anita will agree to pay private health insurance for the child

- Anita will not require me to pay any child support unless I offer the money myself."

Anita read through the points again in her mind. He was thorough; she had to admit. And most conditions sounded acceptable.

"Ok, I agree with all the points in the legal guardianship point. Health insurance is a no brainer and you won't be liable for any child support payments if you're giving up your rights, but for your peace of mind, I'm happy to leave the points there. I'm also happy to write a will with you getting the legal guardianship if something happens to me. That's not a problem. It makes sense that the child goes to you. But, ... I want to discuss the visiting rights."

George tapped his fingers on the table.

"It's nothing major. I only want to clarify a few things. I would like the agreed visits to be at my house with me present, at least for the first few years. Then, maybe from the age of six, as you said yourself, the visits could happen at your place, or places we agree on."

Anita glanced at George, who nodded.

"Yes, I agree."

She wrote the adjustments in.

"Regarding the day long trips, I would like them to happen at a time AND place agreed on by both of us. And at your cost, of course. And the same would apply to the yearly holidays. Those should happen at a time and place agreed on by both of us, for no longer than a week and again at your cost. The special occasions point is absolutely fine with me. Do you agree?"

"I was definitely counting on paying for the trips, so that's fine. And I'm happy to discuss the place with you. Granted, you'll need to know where your child is at all times. I would like to change the no longer than a week to no longer than a fortnight for the yearly holidays, though. If I ever wanted to take the child overseas, a week wouldn't be enough. What do you think?"

Anita didn't even have a child yet, but already struggled with the prospect of the child being away from her for two whole weeks every year. Wasn't that excessive? Although it wouldn't happen for the first few years, would it? Oh, she just didn't know. She wished Zara was there to advice on the best compromise?

"I'm afraid two weeks of holidays every year sounds too much," said Anita. "Will you accept a condition of the yearly holiday being one week, unless it is an overseas holiday, which can be two weeks? But an overseas holiday will not happen more often than once every three years?"

She studied George's face. "Or more often if we both agree," she added.

George reflected on this condition. "Ok, I guess."

"Perfect," Anita clapped her hands with glee, relief spreading through her body.

"Oh, we're at the library. I shouldn't be this loud," she said, folding her hands in her lap, looking around innocently, but with a pleased expression on her face.

George smiled. "Do you still have time this afternoon? I've got nothing else planned, so we could try to find a lawyer who's free now."

"Yes, great idea."

Anita jumped up and darted for the exit, with George in the tow.

After visiting three law offices near the library, they were no further to their goal. The lawyers were all booked up for the next two weeks or longer. At least, they both had already called their doctors and had scheduled appointments within the next two days, so the test results should be back by the time Anita started ovulating. However, they needed to have the legal agreement signed before their first attempt. Anita didn't want to risk getting pregnant without it. What if George refused to sign it afterwards and then be left with legal guardianship? No, it had to be done first.

"I'm pretty sure there are lawyers on High Street, too. Why don't we check?" Anita suggested.

They walked the short walk to High Street and spotted a solicitor's office.

"I'm sorry, but none of our solicitors are available right now. I can, however, make an appointment for another day. Let me see."

The receptionist searched through the online calendar. "We've got an available appointment next week on Monday, at 1pm. Does that suit?"

Monday was still well before Anita's ovulation day. She would have to take the afternoon off work, but that shouldn't be an issue.

"I can't do that; I cannot take time off on Monday afternoon. You have nothing in the morning, do you?" George enquired.

"I'm sorry, Anita, I've got classes most afternoons."

"I've got Tuesday 9am. Would that be better?" the receptionist asked.

"It works for me," said Anita. "What about you?" she turned to George.

"Yes, perfect."

"Good. What are you needing to have done? So I know how much time to reserve for you."

Anita didn't want to discuss the details with the receptionist, but they had to tell her something.

"Well, I need a will. And then an agreement between the two of us regarding a private matter."

"Ok, the time will depend on the complexity of the will

and the agreement. I will schedule you in for two hours and if it's not enough, you'll have to make another appointment afterwards."

"Yes, that sounds good."

"Great, we will see you on Tuesday at 9am. Have a lovely rest of your day," said the receptionist after recording their names in her computer.

"Well, that's it for now," said George once they walked back into the street.

"Yes, it is. By Tuesday, we might already have the check-up results back, so we could do the first try on Friday or Saturday. I won't know the day exactly until it comes, but I'll let you know as soon as I can."

Anita looked at George with an excited expression. "I am so happy about this. Thank you for coming on board."

"You're welcome. I want to have a child and this feels like a win-win for both of us. I'll see you on Tuesday. Call me if you come up with anything you want to discuss in the meantime and I'll do the same. Goodbye," he said, turning to leave.

"Goodbye, George," Anita replied and set for home.

Her mind buzzing with excitement and happiness, she caught herself skipping. *Oh no, people are staring at me,* she thought. *But who cares? I'm so happy.*

CHAPTER 12

Anita's check-up went well. The doctor said that everything looked good, and she was healthy. She had her regular smear test done a few months prior, with the results still valid. However, she had to have a blood and urine samples sent to the laboratory to test, especially for transmittable and sexual diseases. The results could take up to five days, the doctor said, so she should know by Wednesday next week. Despite the tight timeline, Anita felt relieved that they would still come back before her ovulation time. Although, she felt a bit worried about the results. She could have quite easily caught something nasty during her escapades in London.

"You are looking well, Ms Wright," the doctor commented. "How are you?"

"I'm great. Having the donor has injected me with a new will to live."

"Good. I hope you'll become pregnant. This is a much

safer way to approach the issue. I'm actually curious to follow your journey."

"I'm glad you agree," Anita admitted. "I was so stupid. This time we're both having health checks and we're also signing a legal agreement. We want to have all the bases covered."

"Good. I wish you all the best. We'll let you know the results as soon as they come in. Have a nice day."

Anita thanked him, holding two health reports, one for George and one for work. They had agreed to get a written report from their doctors to give to each other, as well as sharing the test results.

Anita rushed back to work. She had to take time off for the appointment, which wasn't ideal, but it had to be done. At work, Anita blamed her absence on health issues. The doctor had given her a report for her manager stating this without disclosing the actual issue. Anita didn't want to lie, but she found it easier this way. People ask fewer questions when health is involved. Well, it was kind of true anyway and nobody needed to know the real reason.

And now, another waiting game. The last few years had all been a huge waiting game. She waited for clinics to send her the decline letters; she waited for her ovulation days to go to London, and she waited for pregnancy test results. After her attack, she waited to get better. She waited for Zara's wedding and for Zara to come back from her honeymoon. She waited for George's decision and now she was waiting for more results and the legal appointment. And that won't be the end. She will wait for more ovulation times and more pregnancy test results. And if she gets pregnant, she'll have to wait for the first scan and if it's ok, the birth of her child. But that outlook was joyful, so joyful Anita's heart ached. All this waiting will be worth it in the end. It must be.

Anita's entire body relaxed when she spotted George reading real estate notices in the shop window next to the solicitors' office. She didn't even realise how tense she was. Pushing away the little doubt sitting at the back of her mind about him backing out at the very last minute, she walked up to him.

"Are you buying a house?" she said jovially.

"No. I'm good. Good morning. Are you ready?"

"Good morning, I am. Shall we go in?"

Anita led the way into the office.

The same receptionist welcomed them. "Good morning. 9 o'clock appointment, correct? Mrs Cavanagh will be with you shortly; she's one of our most experienced solicitors. You are in expert hands. You can wait for her over there," she said, pointing at a waiting area beside the window.

They didn't have to wait long before a grey-haired woman walked to them.

"Ms Wright and Mr Pearce, I presume? Welcome, my name is Lorraine Cavanagh. Please, follow me into my office."

After offering them a cup of tea, she asked, "How can I help you today?"

"Well, we are planning to have a baby, but ..." Anita set to explain their issue in detail, not sure how the lawyer would react.

The lawyer listened to her and then said in a matter of fact, "Yes, a legal agreement in this case is a great idea. It will protect both of you and the child as well. Do you have any specific details you want included?"

Anita, relieved the lawyer didn't judge her, pulled out a sheet of paper with the points she and George had agreed on. She had rewritten them to include all the changes they had made.

The lawyer read it carefully. "You've done a thorough job; you've clearly considered all the possibilities."

"That was George," Anita had to admit.

"Yes," said George, "I wanted to make sure I will have regular contact with the child."

"I see that. And you are ok with everything written here, Ms Wright?"

Anita nodded.

"Ok, I would like to clarify a few points with you. You both talk about a child, however, there is a chance you will end up with more children than one. You could have multiples at this time, or you could decide in the future to have another child or children together. I would recommend you to specify that this agreement relates to all the future children, not only this one. Do you agree?"

Yes, they both agreed. Neither of them had considered this previously, but Anita straight off started imagining what her life would be like with more children than just one. She had always wanted a child and now her mind filled with the word 'children' and she couldn't get it out. How incredible would it be to give the first baby a sibling later on? She would be the happiest mother ever.

"Regarding Ms Wright's will," the solicitor continued, pulling Anita back to reality. "We can write the will today and specify that it applies to all the future children you might have, either with Mr Pearce or with someone else. We could also write the will after you become pregnant and you know you will be having a child. I wouldn't recommend doing it any later, in case something happens to you during pregnancy or childbirth. Your child's and Mr Pearce's rights wouldn't then be protected. What do you prefer?"

"I want to do the will today."

Anita turned to George. "What about you? It was your condition."

"Yes, today makes the most sense."

"Very well. Let's get to work then. We've got quite a bit of ground to cover?"

Mrs Cavanagh sat behind her computer. "I've got a form for you to fill in, Ms Wright, with the information for your will."

She printed a form out and gave it to Anita. "While you are doing this, I will draft the agreement."

Anita bent over the form, filling in the first simple questions—her name, date of birth, address and occupation.

The following questions were trickier. Did she wish to be buried or cremated? Well, she had never thought about this before. What did she actually want? The vision of fire consuming her body wasn't pleasant. However, the image of her body under the ground with maggots, bugs and mice crawling through it brought shivers to her spine. She circled cremated and moved on.

Who will be the executor of the will? She filled in Zara's name and details. Zara would agree.

What about an alternative executor? Anita didn't have anyone else to write in that line. She was the only child and her parents had passed away. Her grandparents had also gone, but she was sure they wouldn't be acceptable executors given their age, anyway. She didn't have any aunts or uncles and therefore no cousins. And she wouldn't trust any of her other friends with her life. What to do? Was she allowed to write an unborn child in the will? Well, why not? That might work. She filled it in. The lawyer would advise if it couldn't be done.

Next question. Who will be the guardian of your child/children? Here she wrote George's details, adding that this was only for the child/children fathered by George. She wrote Zara's name for the other children; in case she had any.

Like that I will, Anita thought.

Did she wish to gift anything specific, either assets or money, to anyone? No, not really, she owned nothing special, no special inherited jewellery or similar. Her personal chattels and estate were to be left to her children, and if they didn't survive her, to Zara Howard.

At what age would she like her estate to be distributed to her children? Well, when they were adults, and knew how to deal with it for sure. 21 seemed young. Maybe 25 rather? They could wait a few years if necessary. *Yes, 25 sounds better.*

Anita scanned her answers again. *Yes, that should do.* The lawyer had her nose buried in the computer still and George was reading a magazine. She also picked up a magazine and flicked through the pages, not really interested in anything in it.

In about 10 minutes, Mrs Cavanagh glanced up from the screen. "Oh, you're finished. Great. I'll print out the agreement draft so you both can have a read and, in the meantime, draft your will." She pulled a stack of papers from the printer, giving them a copy each.

Skimming Anita's form, she said, "This is all good. Have a thorough read through the agreement draft and make any changes you want. Once it is all typed up and signed, it will become legally binding, so make sure you agree with everything written there." Sitting back at her desk, she left them to it.

Anita studied the draft. The agreement points were laid out exactly the way they had wanted them. The lawyer just wrote them all in legal jargon. Why couldn't they be written in plain English? This was so hard to read and Anita had to reread some points several times to understand what they said. Well, obviously it needed to be written like this so that it was legal.

Mrs Cavanagh added one extra point. She wrote that this agreement in no way prevented Anita or George from entering a relationship and having children with someone else. Anita liked it. She wanted to have the freedom to choose should the opportunity arrive.

She pointed it out to George. "Are you ok with this point?"

"Sure," he said. "We don't want to limit our future lives. You never know what might happen."

Anita read the whole document one more time, making sure all the details were correct. Especially those concerning the visiting times George would have their child and the trips. Those were vital. She wanted to allow George regular contact with the child, but she didn't want him to be able to come whenever he wanted to. After all, this will be her baby. As bad as it sounded, he was only a tool to achieving her dream.

"Are you finished? Is everything ok?" Mrs Cavanagh asked.

"Yes, it all looks great," said George.

Anita nodded in agreement.

"Perfect. Here is a draft of your will, Ms Wright. You should review that all the details are correct."

Anita skimmed over the will. The details were identical to those she filled into the form, just full of legal jargon again. Anita showed the part about legal guardianship to George, who nodded in agreement.

"Yes, it looks good."

"Excellent. I'll print out the final copies and invite a colleague to witness the signing of the documents." The printer buzzed to life and spat several sheets of paper out. "I'll be right back."

Anita glimpsed at the clock. They had been in the office for almost two hours. "We should be done within our time slot," she pointed at it.

Mrs Cavanagh came back into the office, followed by a male lawyer. "This is my colleague, John McClinton. He will witness the signing of the documents."

She picked up the documents from the printer. "Please, review your will one more time, Ms Wright, and sign and date it if all correct. Can you please also initial each page, confirming your agreement with the details?"

Anita skimmed the information and initialled, signed, and dated the will. The solicitor added her signature and so did her colleague.

"Now the agreement. Please, review the information again, and initial each page, just like before. And sign and date on the lines below."

Both Anita and George followed the directions and passed it back to the lawyers who did their part.

"All done. Let me put these in envelopes for you and you'll be sorted." She pulled three envelopes from her drawers. On one of them she noted, Will of Ms Anita Wright; and on the other two, Legal Guardianship Agreement between Ms Anita Wright and Mr George Pearce. After inserting the correct documents inside, she passed the envelopes to Anita and George.

"Here are your copies."

"Thank you very much," Anita said while George shook the lawyer's hand.

"Good luck to you both. If you need anything else, please contact me and we can rewrite, adjust or add anything you wish to have added."

Mrs Cavanagh shook Anita's hand in farewell. "The receptionist will send you the invoice shortly."

They thanked her again and left.

Once outside, Anita said, "So, this part is done. How was your check-up?"

"Good, here's the report," he pulled a piece of paper from his pocket.

Anita gave him hers in exchange.

"The test results should be back tomorrow, so I'll call you when I get them."

"Mine are not back either. I'm expecting them today or tomorrow as well. I should be ovulating on Friday or

Saturday, so hopefully we'll have all the results by the end of the week."

"Ok, I have to run now. I've got afternoon classes to teach," said George.

"I have work as well. Have a lovely day, George," Anita said. "And thank you."

CHAPTER 13

Anita's test results came back the very afternoon - all clear. A gush of relief swept over her. Given the unknown history of the men she had sex with in London, the results could have shown anything. She forwarded the message to George. A reply soon came, thanking her.

The next day at lunchtime, Anita's phone beeped. George's results were clear too. Her body tensed, a shiver running down her spine. The time had come. She sent a message back:

> Brilliant, thank you. I'll let you know when I'm ovulating, prob Friday or Saturday

On Friday morning, Anita had raised basal temperature and more of a discharge. She knew these signs well.

> I'm ovulating. Can you come tonight?

> Yes. I can be at yours at 7

> Perfect. See you then

Anita put the new menstrual cup she had bought especially for these pregnancy attempts into a sanitising solution. She really didn't want to use her old one. Her hands shook while getting it ready.

Why am I so nervous? she asked herself. *It will be ok. I should be excited and not nervous. Compared to what I've been through, this will be easy. Weird, but easy.*

"Zara!" Anita called her friend on the way to work. "I'm ovulating. We're going to try tonight."

"Awesome. Do you want me to come?" Zara offered.

"Umm ..., I don't think so," Anita said. "It will be weird enough without you being present. I'm quite nervous, to be honest, and I'm sure we would both be even more embarrassed if anyone else was in the house."

"Fair enough. I have to run now. Good luck tonight and call me afterwards."

"I will. Have a good day."

George arrived at 7pm on the dot. Anita opened the door, more nervous than ever. She had tried everything possible to control her mind, with no luck. George walked in, avoiding eye contact.

"Are you nervous?" Anita asked.

"Terribly. What if I can't ... hmm ... perform?" he finally said.

"If it helps you, I can't stop shaking. Do you want a cup of tea or rather get started?"

"Let's get through this as soon as possible. The longer we wait, the more nervous I'll be."

"I agree. The spare room is upstairs."

Anita led George into the bedroom she set up for him. She had rinsed the cup after taking it out of the solution earlier and laid it beside a box of tissues and a towel on the bed.

"I'm not sure what else you need, but this is the cup I'll be inserting in, so please try to get as much as possible inside."

"I'll do my best," George grinned.

"I'll be in my bedroom across the hall. Call me when it's ready. I need to insert it straight away. Well, I suppose I'll leave you to it then."

Anita walked to her bedroom. Picking up a book, she tried to read. Three pages later, she had no idea what she had just read. With a moan, she threw it down on the bed. Strolling to the window, she watched the sky outside, but she needed a better distraction than a few flittering birds. The phone! Anita scrolled through her social media but nothing took her mind off the happenings in the next room.

Oh, how great it would be to be a fly on the wall to see what he is doing, she thought. *No! Wait! It wouldn't, not really. I don't want to see that!*

Anita checked the time, 7.42pm. *What's taking him so long? He must be having issues.* No surprise there, she wouldn't be able to do much under pressure either.

Anita heard the door opening. In her eagerness to get there, she banged her shin hard on the corner of the bed. Hissing in pain and swearing under her breath, she rushed out of her room.

"Here you go," said George.

Anita grabbed the cup and flew into the bathroom. Sitting above the toilet, she tried to manoeuvre the cup inside. This proved to be no simple feat. She had never needed to insert it with liquid already inside. And it grossed her out as well.

Come on, how do I do this? Oh no, it's leaking, yuck. Argh, how will I ever get it in? This is impossible, Anita swore.

She spent ages trying to fold it in a way that wouldn't spill its contents. Finally, the cup opened inside. *What a mission.*

She scrubbed her hands, trying to get all the spills off.

Anita found George leaning against the balustrade, waiting for her.

"You can go downstairs and have a cup of tea if you'd like. I want to lie down for a bit to help the sperm swim upwards. What if otherwise they just sit in the cup and do nothing?"

"All good."

"Help yourself to some biscuits in the tin on the table as well. And there are magazines on the rack," Anita called after him.

She flopped on the bed, stuffing lots of pillows underneath her bottom and resting her legs against the wall. *I should stand upside down, but this will have to do. How long should I stay like this?* she wondered. *10 or 20 minutes? I'll call Zara in the meantime.*

"It's done," she chirped when Zara picked up the phone. "I'm currently lying on the bed with my legs up the wall and pillows underneath my bum. If someone was watching me, they would have to laugh."

"Sounds fun. I hope it works. So, how did it go?"

"Well, we'll know soon enough, but what a pain to get the cup inside. I couldn't fold it, so the sperm wasn't leaking out. If it doesn't work, we'll have to try the syringe method next. The cup is so tedious. I can only imagine George aiming into it."

Zara laughed at the other end. "Oh yes, it is not big, that's true. A bigger container will be easier next time, but hopefully, you don't need a next time. Fingers crossed you get pregnant straight away. Wouldn't that be absolutely amazing?"

"Yes, that would be wonderful. The next two weeks will be so long. I know that already."

"Where is George now? Did he go home?"

"No, I sent him downstairs to have a cup of tea and biscuits. What you reckon? Is 20 minutes enough? I don't want to rush it, but I don't want to stay like this forever."

"Even 10 should be fine, I would think. You just need to get the swimmers out of the cup. Once inside, they'll know what to do. At least, you would hope so."

Zara laughed again, with Anita joining in.

"I'll go downstairs now. Thanks, Zara. I'll see you tomorrow? Do you still want to go shopping?"

"For sure, shall we go to Reading? I need some new boots, and I haven't seen anything I like here in Maidenhead."

"Sounds good. I'll pick you up around 10 then. Have a great night."

"You too, and good luck to your swimmers," Zara chuckled again.

Anita put down the phone, still smiling. She walked downstairs and discovered George reading a magazine, an empty cup beside him and the tin of biscuits opened.

"How did you go?" he said.

"Tricky. Do you want another cup? I mean a cup of tea, not a menstrual one. I definitely need one," said Anita, rolling her eyes.

"No, I'll head home. It's been quite the evening," George winked; composed once again.

"It definitely has. Thanks for coming. I'll be in touch," said Anita, walking him to the door.

CHAPTER 14

"No! No! No! No! No!" cried Anita, tears streaming down her face.

Bugger, bugger, bugger ... breathe, just breathe, she thought. *You knew the chances of you getting pregnant straight away were slim. You'll try again. It's ok, calm down. Nothing is lost yet. You'll try again next month. And the next, until it works. And it will work. It must.*

Composed again, Anita had to talk to Zara.

"I got my period," said Anita when Zara answered the phone.

"I'm so sorry, hun. Are you ok?"

"Yes, I'm fine. But I must admit that I had a little cry ..., and a shout."

"That's ok. Are you feeling much better for it? I always scream all my emotions out into the world. It helps me to deal with them."

Anita giggled, "True, I'm much better. I needed a good

shout. With so much pressure inside, the scream released some of it out."

"You'll try again, won't you?"

"Oh yes, we'll continue trying until I get pregnant. Or until George gets sick of it. If it happens, I'll need another man. Oh god, I don't want to hunt for another man. This was hard enough. And ... I like George. I think he would be a great father."

Now it was Zara's turn to laugh. "Well, this is something I have never ever expected you to say."

"Say what?"

"That you like a man."

"Oh, you know what I mean. Don't be silly. Nothing romantic is going on."

"I know. I'm sorry. It sounds so odd coming from your mouth. Have you told him already?"

"No, I wanted to talk to you first," admitted Anita. "I'll let him know now."

"Do. We'll talk later. See ya."

Anita stared at her phone. Should she call George? She didn't really want to talk to him. No, a message would have to do. It's not like she's giving him good news, is it? His reply was instant:

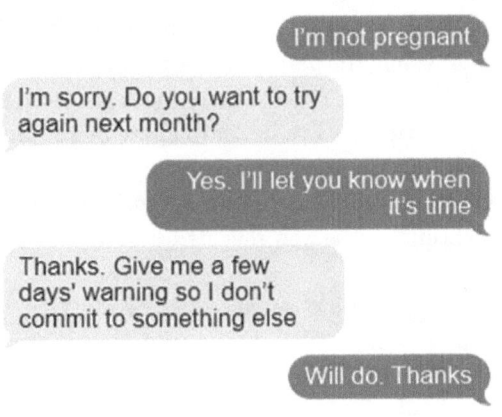

How could buying a simple syringe turn into such a mission? All the shops Anita had tried had none, and they looked at her as if she was a drug addict when she asked about it.

"I promise you I'm not a drug addict; I don't want it for myself," she told one pharmacist, who raised her eyebrows at her. "You know that it is easier to give a child a medicine using a syringe, right?"

Anita lied about the reason, but she couldn't tell them that she needed it to inject sperm into her vagina, could she? The looks that would produce from the other shoppers, or rather the amused and horrified faces of the shop assistants. What a show. She would soon be the talk of the town. Needless to say, she didn't discover one place selling syringes and went home empty-handed.

Once at home, Anita sat at the computer to check online. She searched through heaps of online retailers with no luck. Nobody was selling them. *How hard can this be?* she thought. *Why cannot you buy a simple plastic syringe? It's not like I want to buy needles to go with it as well. Then I would understand. How ridiculous.*

At the end, Anita ordered children's medicine, which included a syringe. While she was at it, she got two different ones, a pain relief and a colic relief. The syringes inside were different. Maybe one would work better than the other. One said it was 5 ml while there was no information for the other one. Would 5 ml be enough? How much sperm does a man ejaculate? A quick internet search revealed that usually not more than 5 ml.

Good, these syringes should be fine, then. Unless George is abnormal, Anita giggled.

"Look, I'm getting ready already," said Anita, showing the bottles of the children's medicines to Zara a few days later.

"I would never expect to have such issues when buying a syringe. Well, I suppose these will come in handy in the future." Anita stored the bottles back into the cupboard.

"Yes, they will. But," Zara smirked, "I suppose you won't want to use the same syringes then."

She pulled a face, and they both laughed. "No, I will not want to give my child medicine from a syringe I used to make them. How gross. Gosh, I'm getting goosebumps just picturing it." Anita shook. "Zara, now you put this image into my mind, I can't unsee it."

Zara's eyes twinkled. "I'm sure you'll forget about it soon enough."

"Yes, until I need to give the kid the medicine. Zara," Anita slapped her forehead dramatically, "you are evil."

"Yep, that's my secret superpower."

"When are you ovulating again?" Zara asked after Anita had made them a cup of tea.

"Probably Sunday. George has free evenings Saturday to Monday and if things go according to plan, we'll try again. Hopefully, we'll both be much calmer for the second attempt. Maybe I was too anxious and the sperm just couldn't enter my egg."

"No, that can't be it. You were distraught after your attack and still got pregnant. That shouldn't make any difference, but then, you never know."

"Exactly, you never know. The syringe should at least imitate the natural movement. I will have to shoot it with some force so it has enough speed to reach the egg."

Anita snorted, "If somebody listened to us, they would say we're crazy."

"Because we are. Do you know anyone else who had gone through this?"

"Well, no, but we're not telling anyone either. None of our other friends know what is happening."

"True," said Zara. "Oh well, never mind. It will be worth it in the end. I can't wait to be an auntie."

"I hope you don't end up being an ancient auntie. And what about my auntiehood? What's happening with you and Chris? Have you started trying yet?"

"Nah, we will wait another year or so. I'm not ready. Chris probably is, but I'm enjoying my freedom at the moment. So, you need to get pregnant soon. I need to know what it is like to be an auntie first."

"Hold on, hold on. I don't need any more pressure on me. It's hard enough as it is."

"I know. And I'm here for you. Don't take me seriously. Chris and I want to wait until we have the house sorted. It's difficult living in a half-finished house. I can't even imagine having a child crawling or running through it on top of everything. That would be a complete nightmare. It's definitely not safe at the moment, even we walk around some areas carefully. You know that."

"Yes, that's true."

Zara and Chris bought an old house. It seemed ok at the beginning, but once they had begun the renovations, they discovered heaps of issues. What they initially considered a little easy project turned into a major undertaking. Zara often said it would be better to ball it down and build a brand new house if only they didn't love the house so much. It had a lot of character and, once renovated, will be a beautiful home. But the renovation was certainly a labour of love on their part.

"Zara, my offer still stands. If you need, I can give you some money towards it."

Zara looked at her. "I know. We'll keep it in mind. For now, we're happy to work on one thing at a time. We're in no rush. It is liveable, just not that pleasant. It will be ok, don't worry. As long as we have a roof above our heads, we'll be fine."

"But if it meant you can't have a baby yet ..." Anita left the sentence hanging.

"Honestly, Anita, I'm fine. My biological clock is not ticking; it is standing very still. I know if it happened, I would be thrilled, but if it happens in two or three-years' time, I won't mind at all."

"Good. I want you to be happy. You've helped me more than I can ever repay."

"Oh, don't mention it. That's what friends are for, aren't they?" Zara smiled. "You would do the same for me."

"Yes, I would." Anita reached across the table and squeezed Zara's hand. "Thank you."

CHAPTER 15

"I'll be back soon," said George, shutting the door to the spare bedroom.

Anita waited in her room, wondering how he was getting on with the new measuring cup she had bought. It was one of those cups schools used for science experiments; she even remembered using it. It was narrow at the bottom and wider on the top, with a wide stand; and it certainly looked easier to aim into.

As if I know what he has to do, right? she giggled. *Well, at least I didn't have to give him anything from the kitchen. No, this cup is going to be a dedicated baby making cup. A sperm cup,* Anita giggled again. *This time, we're both much more composed. By the time we do it the tenth time, I'll be all good,* she thought. *But please, don't take so long, my future baby.*

The door opened, with George giving her the cup. "This is still so weird, isn't it?"

"I know. I can't get used to it either. Can you hold the cup steady please? I need to suck the sperm into the syringe."

Anita concentrated, trying to get every last bit.

"Done." She showed him victoriously and disappeared into her bedroom.

The measuring line read just over 3.5 ml. *So, George isn't abnormal,* chortled Anita.

She spread her legs on the bed and inserted the syringe inside. Holding it with both hands, she squirted the contents in as fast as she could. With her legs up against the wall and cushions underneath her bottom, she stayed still again, listening to George boiling water for tea in the kitchen and opening the tin of biscuits.

Good thing I topped up the chocolate-covered biscuits, she thought. *He liked them last time and I don't blame him; they are tasty. And now I want one. How long has it been? 15 minutes. That should be enough.*

Anita walked to the kitchen and sat at the opposite side of the table. "How did it go this time? Easier?"

"Oh yes, I wasn't as nervous for sure, so it went a bit faster; and the larger cup is better. Much easier to aim into, if you need to know."

Anita chuckled, "I'm glad. To be honest, I found tonight much better, too. It was hard to insert the menstrual cup with the sperm inside; it kept on leaking out. This was easy. Just shoot, and all done."

After a moment of silence, Anita asked the question sitting on her mind since their first attempt. "If it doesn't work again, are you happy to keep going?"

"Yes, I am."

George stirred his tea, obviously contemplating something. "I should tell you the truth, Anita. You told me about your history, so you've got the right to know about mine. I had always planned on my partner and I adopting a child. After he told me he never actually wanted to have one, and that he didn't know how much it meant to me, I didn't know what to do. He suggested I find another man because he wasn't the one for me. That hurt. And it still does."

George's voice trembled. "I left Spain because I couldn't be anywhere near him. The pain almost tore me apart, and I gave up on the dream of becoming a father. By the time I would have met and fallen in love with another man, I would be too old for a child. And then life threw you into my path. I know it will not be the same as having a child full time, but ..., this child will be mine, truly mine, and that changes a lot; it makes all the difference. So yes, I'm happy to keep trying until we succeed."

"Thank you for sharing, George. The conditions in the agreement are at our discretion. So, if the circumstances allow, you'll be able to spend more time with the child than it says. A fatherly figure is important." Anita surprised herself in saying that. How did she get there? She didn't want a father in her child's life. She didn't want a man in hers. What had changed? Why was she ok with him playing a bigger part than they had agreed on? She didn't understand her own mind.

"Thank you. Are you ok if I call it the night?" George interrupted her train of thoughts.

"Of course, it's getting late, anyway. I'll be in touch. Good night."

George let himself out of Anita's house. She stayed sitting, staring into her cup, processing her own thoughts and feelings and what George had told her.

He had been through a lot of disappointment, just like her. How long did Zara say he was together with his partner? 13 years? Maybe 15? Anita couldn't remember. *But to learn after so many years that your partner is not on the same page in such a critical matter must be devastating. No wonder he wanted to come back home; I wouldn't want to stay there either. No wonder I feel bad for him. That must be it. I'm just feeling bad for him. It will pass. Well, let's make both of our dreams come true, at least to some extent in his case.*

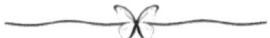

"Not again," Anita whined at the sight of blood. She had known since the morning her period was coming; the pressure and the warmth in her stomach were the telltale signs. Still, she had hoped for the rest of the day that the signs were fake.

Anita recorded the second failed attempt in her diary. In the next months, these records had, to her despair, multiplied:

Attempt #1: menstrual cup, time - evening
Result: failure

Attempt #2: first syringe, time - evening
Result: failure

Attempt #3: second syringe, time - evening
Result: failure

Attempt #4: second syringe, time - morning
Result: failure

Attempt #5: first syringe, time - morning
Result: failure

After this attempt, Anita's period came five days late, much heavier and with strong cramps. *Way to give me a flicker of hope,* Anita sniffled. But at the back of her mind, she knew this attempt was not a complete failure, but a very early miscarriage. Her periods were never this heavy and never this late. It meant that both she and George could have children, and knowing that meant a lot.

Attempt #6: first syringe, time - midday
Result: failure

Anita sat in the classroom at the nursery, watching the children drawing and writing their letters to Santa. The end of November brought much colder weather to England, and the darkness crept in earlier. As the children worked on their letters, Anita picked up a piece of paper to write her own.

Dear Santa,

I promise I have been very good this year. I'm sorry about last year. I certainly didn't deserve any presents after my appalling behaviour.

I know you cannot give me what I'm going to ask for, but I don't know who else to ask anymore. If by any chance you can grant me a wish, I would love to get pregnant. I promise to be always good and look after the baby well.

Yours,
Anita Wright

Anita sensed being watched and looked up to a smiling face of a little 5-year-old boy, Joel, peering at her.

"Are you writing a letter to Santa, Miss Wright?"

"Yes, I am, Joel. Have you finished yours?"

"Yep, I'm all done. What did you wish for?" Joel enquired.

"I'm not sure you're supposed to tell people what you wish for."

"Yes, you can. Santa doesn't care. Everyone knows I want a new bike and I've been good, so Santa will bring me one for sure."

"What a great present to wish for, Joel. I guess Santa can't bring me what I wish for, anyway."

"Well, why did you ask for a present Santa can't bring?"

"Because I don't know who else to ask."

"You have to ask the person who can give it to you, you know? Who is it?"

"Well, it's not that simple, but I suppose it would be nature. And I really can't ask nature, can I?"

"Nature is like trees and grass and flowers, right?"

"Yes, correct. Nature is all the life surrounding us, basically everything people didn't make. So, trees, grass, flowers, but also rivers and seas, mountains and rocks, as well as most of the food we eat."

"Well, then you can definitely ask it. You just have to climb up a tall hill and shout your wish into the nature. But really loud, you know? So it hears you. Try it, I'm sure it will work!" said little Joel with an all-knowing face before running off to play.

Anita thought about this. *And I'm going to do just that. I'm going to climb up a mountain and shout into the world my wish to have a baby. I've tried everything else so this can't hurt.*

She walked over to Joel. "Thank you for the advice, Joel. I'll climb up a mountain this weekend and ask Mother Nature to grant me my wish. Thank you."

"You're welcome, Miss. Anytime."

Anita grinned from ear to ear at this. *What a child.*

"Are you up for a little climb?" Anita called George in the evening.

During the last few months, the two of them had spent a lot of time together and had become close. They talked after each attempt for several hours and went for teas and walks together. They had found that they had lots of similar hobbies and likes. Anita had never dreamed of having a good relationship with a man before. The possibility of the male wanting something more at some stage prevented that. But with George, she knew it wouldn't happen. George was not interested in her as a woman, he liked her as a person, and she liked him in return.

"What do you mean?"

Anita told George what had happened at the nursery. "So, I'm going up Ashley Hill on Saturday to shout my wish into the surrounding forests, and if it doesn't work, I'll climb up Ben Nevis next. Are you coming with me?"

"Do you mean up Ben Nevis? Well, that's quite a trek," George laughed. "But I could probably manage Ashley Hill. Well, is it even a hill? It's more of a knoll, isn't it? But I know of a fantastic little tea room in Henley we could stop at afterwards."

"Sounds like a plan to me. I'll take any hill at this moment, and Ashley Hill is the closest. Shall I pick you up around 10 on Saturday?"

"Yes, can't wait. Let's shout into the forests."

On Saturday morning, Anita stopped in front of George's apartment building. He jumped into the car, wrapped in a warm jacket.

"It's a tad chilly today," he announced.

"Yes, it is. I've brought a flask of hot tea."

"Good thinking."

They drove to Hurley and parked by the curb on High Street. The crisp air bit Anita's cheeks the moment she got out of the car. Shivering, Anita wrapped her coat tighter around her body. She smelled the coming winter in the light breeze.

"It's much colder here than in Maidenhead. I didn't expect such a huge difference."

"Yes, we are higher."

"I've done this walk a few times before; it is nice," said Anita to George. "It shouldn't take us more than two to three hours."

"Oh good, it's too cold for a longer walk."

"Don't worry, you'll soon warm up. I can't believe you're such a couch potato."

"A couch potato?" George's eyes grew wide with exaggeration. "I'm not a couch potato. I just don't like the cold."

"You'll be fine for once. Ready?"

Anita led the way. They both warmed up in no time, and Anita chuckled when George undid the top of his jacket. "Warm enough yet?"

They didn't rush, and they didn't talk.

How good to be out in nature in good company, thought Anita. She was enjoying the walk immensely. She loved the comfortable quiet between them, with neither of them feeling the need to talk. Once they entered the forest, fog curled around their feet while the trees and bushes above stood clear of it.

"Isn't it like magic?" Anita whispered, stopping to admire the view.

By the time they reached the summit, or as close to it as possible, droplets of sweat dripped down Anita's back. George's cheeks were flushed, his hat in his hand and gloves stuffed in the pockets.

"Only a few people are out today," Anita remarked. "Normally, you meet lots."

"Well, who would want to trek in such cold?"

"You don't look cold," she grinned. "But it's so beautiful today. It's true that I've never done the walk this late in the year. Oh well, I don't mind, at least nobody is here and nobody will hear us shouting. Speaking of which, I think this place is as good as any."

"Are you honestly going to shout into the wild?"

"Well, that's why I came here. Aren't you?"

"I don't know. Isn't it, well, odd?"

"I don't care. If there is even the slightest chance it might work, I'm up for it. I'll happily do it just for the fun. Watch me. Here I go." Anita took a deep breath, "NATURE! CAN I PLEASE HAVE A BABY? PLEASE, HELP ME GET PREGNANT!"

"Wow, it felt good to let it out. I'll go again. Join me."

George stood beside her, amused. "You really meant it. Ok, here goes nothing."

This time they shouted together. "NATURE! CAN WE PLEASE HAVE A BABY?"

"I'll go again," said Anita. "I WISH TO HAVE A BABY."

"I WISH MY SPERM TO IMPREGNATE THIS LADY BESIDE ME."

Anita burst into fits of laughter. "Well ..., that ... would have ... done it."

"Yep, it's sorted. Our wish is sure to get granted now. I'm ready for a cup of tea."

"Here's the flask."

George wrinkled his nose. "I want something proper. And a nice plate of scones."

"Scones do sound good. I'm sold."

CHAPTER 16

Attempt #7: first syringe, time - evening
Result: not known yet, period due 28th December

"I still can't get over this kitchen. You've done such a great job, you two," said Anita, getting a potato salad ready in Zara and Chris's new kitchen on Christmas Eve. "I feel like I'm cooking on one of the telly shows."

"I know. Would you believe that three months ago, there was a hole in the wall over there?" said Zara, pointing at a wall now covered in green splashback tiles.

"What a surprise find that was," Chris joined in with a chuckle. "I never expected to uncover an enormous hole behind the pantry."

"If at least it was filled with treasure, I wouldn't mind," said Zara, "but it was only rubbish; just stones, bits of wood, and bricks."

"It might have been messy then, but it turned out

beautiful in the end. I just love this island, it's such a great central feature. You've got so much space to prepare food."

Anita ran her finger alongside the smooth surface of the dark granite island, admiring it.

"It's amazing, I must admit, although I might be a bit biased, but this is definitely my favourite room in the house at the moment. I could spend the whole day here. If only the rest of the house was already done too."

"It won't take long, Zara. You're halfway there."

"I know, and it's actually quite fun making the house the way we want it. I'm enjoying it."

"I'll get it," said Chris as the doorbell rang.

"Is someone else coming for dinner?"

"Oh, didn't I tell you? We invited George as well. I hope you don't mind."

Anita shook her head. "Not at all. It will be good to have him here."

"You've been spending more time with him, haven't you?" Zara winked at Anita.

"I like him."

"Well, here we go again. Anita Wright likes a man."

"Yes, it's nice to have a male friend who is easy to talk to and wants nothing of me."

"Just a baby," Zara pointed out.

"That's mutual."

"Merry Christmas," bellowed George, walking into the kitchen.

"Merry Christmas to you."

"I say, you've done a great job at this kitchen, Chris and Zara. You could photograph it for a magazine," said George, looking around the room.

"Thank you. We love how it turned out," Chris agreed.

"Ok, Chris said to bring a desert, but I didn't know what to get, so I hope this is adequate. I've got a fruit cake, custard and ice cream."

"Perfect, cake will finish the dinner off nicely. We've got a roast turkey and vegetables, warm potato salad, boiled broccoli, and Anita insisted on Brussels sprouts. Bleurgh," Zara gagged.

"I like Brussels sprouts. You don't have to eat them," Anita smirked at her friend.

"I won't eat them, don't you worry about that," Zara responded, carrying the serving platters and bowls to the table.

"Wine, anyone?" Chris asked when they were at the table.

Zara and George pushed their glasses forward, but not Anita.

"Not for me, thanks."

"You're not having any?"

"No, my period is due in a few days, so just in case. I don't want to do anything wrong."

"You're too careful, Anita. Having a little glass of wine wouldn't do the baby any harm."

"Maybe, but I will rather not risk it. I'll have some juice, please. And if things don't work out again, I'll have a lot of wine on New Year's Eve. I'll make up for it, you'll see."

"Is that a promise?" winked Zara.

"That's a threat," sneered Anita.

"I'll hold you up to it and join you. Well, Merry Christmas everyone," Zara lifted her glass. "Thank you for coming to celebrate it with us. It is lovely to finally entertain friends in our new home. Now, dig in."

Anita filled up her plate with the delicious food, putting two helpings of the sprouts on.

"I'll have some Brussels sprouts to help Anita out," said George, loading a pile of sprouts onto his plate.

Anita giggled. "You don't have to sacrifice your taste buds on my behalf. I love Brussels sprouts and will happily eat the whole bowl by myself."

"I actually like them," George admitted.

"Good. So, it's only these two crazies who don't."

"Because they're disgusting." Zara screwed up her face to everyone's laughter.

"What are you doing tomorrow?" George asked.

"We're having lunch with my family," said Chris. "I've got three siblings, all with children, so you can imagine how busy the lunch gets."

"It's busy, but always a lot of fun," added Zara. "Chris's family is hilarious ..., and noisy."

"Not too noisy."

"Oh yes, noisy. You've got like ten nieces and nephews now. When they all start, it's craziness."

"True. I can't wait."

"Sounds fun. Where are you having the lunch?" George asked.

"At my parents' house in Windsor," said Chris.

"So, not far to go."

"Which is good," added Zara, "because we have dinner with my grandparents afterwards."

"What about you, Anita? What are you doing tomorrow?"

Anita had nowhere to go. "Well, nothing really. I'll go to the cemetery, watch some movies and eat crisps and ice cream. That's the plan."

"You're going to be alone on Christmas Day?" said George, raising his eyebrows.

"I'm usually alone; I don't mind at all. It's always such a relaxing day. I actually like it."

"If you wanted to," said George in a quiet voice, "you could come with me."

"Where are you going?"

"To my mum's in Suffolk. My sister will be there with her two children as well. It's never as busy as Chris's Christmas sounds, but it's pleasant."

"Thank you for the invitation, but I think I'll pass. How would you introduce me, anyway?" Anita grinned. "Mum, please meet Anita Wright, the woman who I am artificially inseminating."

Zara burst out laughing. "Sounds perfect. You should so do it."

"Well, you've become much more than that in the last months," George's face turned serious.

"I know. I'm sorry. But I will still pass. I like my quiet Christmas."

"Ok, I understand."

Anita saw how disappointed he was. *I'll apologise to him again afterwards,* she decided.

"Shall we have a desert now?" Zara offered, trying to lighten up the mood in the silent and solemn room. "And who wants to watch a fun Christmas movie before heading out to the Midnight Mess? I certainly do. Is anyone else up for it?"

"Sounds like a plan, but I want to eat the whole tub of ice cream first."

Anita loved ice cream; it was one of her guilty pleasures.

"Is that your goal for the night? To eat a whole tub of ice cream?"

"Yep, and I've got another ready at home for tomorrow," said Anita. "It's good to set achievable goals, especially at Christmas time."

CHAPTER 17

28th December, no period.

Anita's period had occasionally been a day early or late, but so far, she hadn't felt any of the usual signs of it coming. *I will not put my hopes up,* she said to herself, remembering the recent one-week long delay.

The last few days had been a complete bliss. Anita spent a lot of time at home, watching telly, eating ice cream and other comfort food. She slept until late in the mornings and stayed up until at least midnight on most of the nights. For Anita, not having to wake up was the best part of holidays. She loved her job, but working with children put a lot of pressure on her emotional well-being.

She met with Zara on Boxing Day for a quick visit, but that was the only time she had seen anyone since their joint Christmas Eve dinner. Zara and Chris were busy with their renovations, hoping to finish the main bathroom by the time Chris had to go back to work after New Year's. And Zara, flitting between her own house and her grandparents, didn't have much time left for catch ups.

George also messaged a few times. Anita knew he cared, but she sensed some pity in his messages. He didn't agree with her spending the Christmas season alone. It seemed like he couldn't even imagine it. Anita didn't mind being alone; she liked it. Christmas was different, but not much. Sure, she would have loved to have a delicious lunch with her parents. She would have loved to get some presents from loved ones and to have a family to buy presents for. Maybe, when she had a child, things would change. For now, a tub of ice cream and great movies on the telly were all she needed for the festive season.

30th December, no period.

"When are you going to do the test, Anita?" George asked in the evening over the phone.

"Tomorrow afternoon. So, if I'm not pregnant, I can drown my sadness in wine, a lot of wine."

"I'm sorry I can't be there," said George, sitting on the train to Edinburgh, where he was going to spend a few days with his friends.

"Umm ..., no worries at all. I think it's better if I do it alone."

Anita wanted to be the only one to know the result, at least for a while. She wanted to celebrate or mourn on her own. She wanted to laugh or scream without the audience.

"Ok, but you'll let me know as soon as you know, promise?"

"Yes, I'll call you straight away." W*ell,* Anita thought, *not straight away, but you don't need to know that. It will be my secret.*

31st December, no period.

At 3pm, Anita plucked up her courage and took a pregnancy test out of the cupboard. She pulled the test strip out of the box, her hands shaking so much in a mixture of anticipation and fear.

"Ok, let's pee on you," she said, walking to the bathroom.

Awkwardly sitting on the toilet, Anita aimed straight at the strip. She counted up the recommended time, "One, two, three, four, five," adding, "six, seven" for good measure. She laid the strip on the basin, and after washing her hands, left the bathroom.

Setting her phone alarm to five minutes, she grouched, "What do I do with myself now?"

Anita, Zara, and Chris were going to a New Year's Eve party. Anita would have much rather stayed at home on this occasion. She enjoyed parties and clubs, but she didn't want to go out that particular day. She would much rather spend the night in front of the telly again.

Oh well, she thought, *quite often when you're not looking forward to something, it turns out great. What should I wear?*

She chose a black top with white flowers and a pair of jeans. Her black flats were downstairs already. It hardly ever snowed in her part of England, but she would still need a warm coat to brave the December night.

The alarm startled Anita. "Oh my, it's time."

She ran to the bathroom, and with her hand on the doorknob, froze. *I don't want to see it. Why didn't I invite Zara over? She could have checked it for me. What if it's negative? Or worse, what if it's positive and I miscarry again? I don't want to go through another miscarriage. I cannot go through another miscarriage. That would kill me. No, it won't happen again. It can't. I won't have another miscarriage. ... Oh, I need to go in. I need to do it now.*

Anita's will pushed her body into the bathroom. Trying not to look at the test, she walked to the basin and lifted it up. With her eyes closed, she moved it to her eye level, scared to open them.

"Ok. One, two, three. Look now!"

A surge of energy and happiness burst through her body. Positive. The test was positive!

"IT IS POSITIVE!" Anita yelled in delight.

"Happy New Year!" every person in the room, including Anita, shouted.

People hugged and kissed, wishing each other all the best for the New Year. Zara embraced Anita in the biggest hug.

"You have the best year of all, my friend. I'm so happy for you right now. This is your year, Anita. Do you understand? This is your year!" Zara blurted out, wobbling on unsteady legs.

Anita knew Zara's tipsy state was her fault. After her positive pregnancy test, Anita danced around the house for almost an hour. The news made her twirl in happiness and she just couldn't stop. She sang and danced with joy before calling George.

"I'm pregnant, George. The test was positive."

"That is the best news, Anita. Honestly, the best ever. I ... I don't know what to do. What do we do now?" he laughed.

"Have a baby," Anita chuckled, unable to hide her joy. "But please don't tell anyone yet! Wait until I'm past the first 12 weeks. I don't want anyone else to know in case I miscarry again."

"Of course, that makes sense, although it will be hard to keep it a secret for so long. I'll come and see you when I get back."

"Happy New Year, George."

"The same to you, Anita. Have a great night."

Oh no, the party tonight. She needed to check the allowed food. Rushing to the computer, Anita typed 'food to avoid in pregnancy'. She had to refresh her memory. After glancing at it when she fell pregnant the first time, she forgot most of it. Reading the list of foods she shouldn't be eating, she whimpered.

What am I going to eat? Pretty much everything is forbidden or not recommended. And more importantly, what am I going to drink? I need to make a wine drinking plan for the night. People at the party will be drinking. They will expect me to drink as well. They all know I like wine. If I don't drink, it will raise suspicion, and I don't want to get into that conversation tonight. Anita reached for her phone.

"Hi hun, how are you doing?" Zara chirped. "Are you almost ready?"

"I've got news, Zara. I'm pregnant."

"Are you sure? You are, right? Amazing. I'm so happy for you. You must be stoked. ... CHRIS! ANITA IS PREGNANT." Chris mumbled something in the background. "Chris says congratulations."

"Thank you so much. It's pretty amazing," said Anita, "but I need to make a plan for tonight. What do I do? I'll be expected to drink, and I don't want people asking questions."

"We'll manage; easy as. I'll help. You can walk around with a glass of wine and tip some of it here and there occasionally. And I will, from time to time, have a sip of yours or swap our glasses. Don't worry, people will think you're drinking; nobody will be any wiser. Easy as."

"Ok, that might work."

"It will work. Don't doubt my plans. They always work, don't they?"

"Always?" said Anita with a chuckle.

"Oh, almost always then. No way it could be such a fiasco as my ad plan. What's the worst that could happen?"

"You get awfully drunk."

"Well, it won't be the first or the last," laughed Zara. "I'll see you soon."

"See you soon, Zara."

With a lighter mind, Anita got ready and went to the party. And as much as she didn't want to come in the first place, she actually enjoyed it. Catching up with people she hadn't seen for ages and chatting away about the old times was a good way to spend the last day of the year.

Eating and drinking did prove challenging. Everyone brought a plate and so lots of trays were arranged on the tables, filled with various finger food and appetizers. Anita made small puff pastry parcels stuffed with vegetables, so she knew those were safe to eat. But the other stuff? She had no idea. Most of the night, she fed on fruit, vegetables, bread, and crisps. A large plate of sushi, which she loved, dominated the table. She whined, knowing that she couldn't touch it. "This is so annoying."

"What did you say?" a voice said behind her.

She turned to face Hannah, her high school classmate. They used to be great friends before Hannah had moved overseas after they graduated.

"Hannah! It's so nice to see you. When did you come back?"

"Hi Anita, I'm visiting family for the holidays. How is life treating you?"

"I'm good. Still the same. How are you doing?"

"Great. I got married last year and we have a 15-month-old. My husband is somewhere around. I'll introduce you later on."

"That's nice. A girl or a boy?"

"Samuel, a boy. He's amazing. We had issues getting pregnant, but at the end managed. It was quite the journey.

If you only knew how hard it can be when you just keep trying and things are not working out."

Hannah shook her head in dismay.

I know, trust me, I know well enough, Anita thought. Aloud, she said, "I'm sorry to hear that, but I'm happy it worked out for you."

"So am I, thanks. What are you drinking? Your glass is empty."

Hannah pointed at the glass in Anita's hand with a little leftover of red wine at the bottom.

"Just red wine."

Anita had disposed of the first glass easily, tipping some of it into the kitchen sink and some into the basin in the bathroom. She hoped that nobody would notice her empty glass and she would get away with it for the rest of the night.

"I'll get you some more."

Hannah fetched a bottle of red and topped up Anita's glass.

"We can't have you thirsty on New Year's Eve."

Bugger, Anita swore under her breath. "Thank you," she said to Hannah.

While Anita and Hannah chatted, Zara danced to them. "Oh Hannah, you're here. What a surprise," said Zara, hugging their old friend. She put her glass, half filled with red wine, beside Anita's one while talking.

"I'm sorry, I have to bounce. There's a friend I need to greet," she chirped, picking up Anita's full glass and running off.

Zara kept on doing that for most of the night. So, it wasn't surprising that once midnight approached, the world around her spun. Drinking for two would do that.

When leaving the party, Zara had to lean on Chris for support.

"I'm sorry, Zara. I didn't mean to get you drunk."

"That's perfectly alright, my friend. It was worth it."

"Will tomorrow be worth it as well, babe?" Chris asked her with a grin.

"Don't you worry a bit, my darling husband. I will be perfectly alright."

"I'll bring you some pizza and ice cream for lunch. How does that sound?" offered Anita.

"Sounds marvellous. See? Anita will bring me pizza and ice cream. I'll be all good."

"I know you will. I'm just teasing you because whenever you drink, you're so miserable afterwards, but pizza and ice cream should make you happy."

"Trust me, this was a necessity. Anita's state is a secret. Sec-ret!" Zara added in a dramatic way, rolling her eyes and giggling.

"Thank you, Zara. I really appreciate what you did for me tonight."

"It wasn't a hard job and I would gladly do it again."

Anita heard Chris mumbling under his breath, "Let's just see what you think tomorrow."

She giggled. She knew Zara would regret all the drinking the next day and so Anita had to do all she could to make her hangover more comfortable. She hugged her friend, wished her a good sleep and left her in Chris's hands.

What a great night, Anita smiled. *And now for the best year ever.*

CHAPTER 18

Where is Zara? She should have been here already. Anita tapped her foot on the floor of the radiology clinic. Her heart pounded in her chest while in her mind she repeated over and over that the scan would be fine. She didn't want to think about her past, instead trying to focus on the present. But her thoughts still kept on returning to the previous scans and the dreaded words 'no heartbeat'. No wonder she found it hard to keep her cool. No, the heartbeat was there. It had to be.

Anita recalled the difficult conversation she had with George earlier in the week. She booked the scan for the afternoon, knowing he would be teaching. She wanted to tell him they had no other appointments available, but she knew he deserved to know the truth. He deserved to know that she didn't want him there.

"What a shame the appointment is in the afternoon. I would have loved to come," George said in disappointment.

"I'm sorry, George. There's not much I can do," said

Anita. "Actually ..., I'm sorry; I don't want to lie to you. The truth is that I don't want you at this appointment."

George frowned at her in surprise.

"I am still getting used to the fact you are so involved. I have never expected the donor to go to any appointments with me, to be by my side for anything, so this is just, umm, a bit too much."

"I'm sorry you feel like this. I'll give you space," said George, clenching his fists.

"I don't want you to be angry with me, George. I just need time to get used to the fact that you are here. If everything is good, I would love for you to come to the 12-week scan. You'll see the baby already and get photos to show your family. This scan is really just to check if the baby is actually there. That's all they'll be doing. Just checking for the foetus's heartbeat."

George still sulked a bit, but his composure had relaxed. "You are right," he said, "I was never supposed to be this involved, and now I am, it's hard to step back. I want to be here for the baby, you know?"

"And you will, but I don't need you to be here for me." There. It was out. Anita's cheeks turned bright red.

"Oh, I see. Right. I'll wait for your call then."

Anita knew how much she had hurt him. She hated doing it, but she didn't need him to be her emotional support. She needed Zara, and now Zara was running late.

At that moment, Zara burst into the waiting room. "I'm sorry I'm late. I got caught up with Grandpa."

"That's ok, I'm still waiting to be seen."

Zara glanced around. "Where's George?"

"He's not coming."

"Why?"

"I don't need him here."

Anita recapped the conversation.

"He's trying to support you," said Zara.

"I know, but that's not his job. His job is to support the child. I am not his responsibility at all," said Anita, getting flustered with both of them. "I don't need a man to help me. I'm perfectly capable of doing this whole baby thing by myself."

"I know you are, Anita. I'm not saying you are not. Yes, it was always supposed to be only you, you are right. Let's forget about George and just concentrate on the scan. Are you nervous?" said Zara to soothe Anita's anger.

Anita stretched her arms forward to show Zara her shaking hands. "And my stomach is tied in knots, on the top of the bloody nausea, and my throat is so tight I can barely swallow."

"It will be ok. You'll see."

"Ms Wright?" the sonographer came into the waiting room.

Anita and Zara jumped up. "Yes," said Anita.

"Please, follow me into room number 3," she pointed at the door at the end of the corridor.

Anita's throat tightened as she was being ushered into the same room in which she had received the first non-viable pregnancy news. She swallowed hard, her feet refusing to move. Zara nudged her forward.

"Let me confirm your details first. You are eight weeks pregnant, due date September 6th," said the sonographer when Anita finally made it into the room.

She nodded.

"Perfect. Please, lie on the bed and uncover your stomach."

Anita did as told, an anxious sensation spreading through her body, starting in her bare belly and making its way into every single part of her shaky self.

"I'll put this gel on your skin first. It will be cold. And then I'll use the scan to look at the embryo. You can watch on the screen above."

Anita clutched Zara's hand.

"There's no need to be scared," the sonographer said, noticing Anita's anxious state. "This is a routine scan. Don't worry, it doesn't hurt."

"I'm not scared of the scan, but I've had bad news on this bed before."

"Oh, I see. I'll check the foetus now then."

She moved the probe in circular motions around Anita's stomach, sliding it from side to side and up and down without talking. Anita squeezed Zara's hand more and more, not noticing Zara wincing in pain.

"If you look here," said the sonographer, pointing at an area on the screen, "this is the embryo. It is exactly the size it is supposed to be for 8 weeks. The heartbeat is here. Can you see it? It's this faint quiver."

Anita couldn't see much, except for a smudge on the screen, quivering a little now and then. "So, are you saying that everything is ok? The baby is ok? The baby is actually there?"

"Yes, it is."

Sense of relief flooded Anita's body, tears of happiness filling her eyes. She released Zara's hand.

"Thank goodness, Anita. I'm so happy for you. And for my hand as well," said Zara with a chuckle, rubbing her sore hand.

Anita looked at her, her face a mix of happiness and confusion.

"You almost crushed my hand," said Zara in explanation.

"Oh, I'm so sorry. I didn't even realise I was squeezing you so hard."

"No, of course you didn't. You were too nervous. It's ok, it's not broken. Just!" giggled Zara.

Anita beamed with delight. She was having a baby. There was a baby in her stomach and it had a heartbeat and was developing well.

"Here are some tissues. You can wipe your stomach now. We are done for today," said the sonographer.

"Thank you."

"You're welcome. We will see you again for your 12-week scan. Keep well and have a good day."

"Thank you. It will be a good day for sure," said Anita, walking out of the door towards the reception area to pay her bill, Zara following close behind.

Once outside, Anita called George. She didn't really expect him to pick up, knowing he was probably in class, but still gave it a go. Even though he would see a missed call from her, she still sent a message as well:

> Everything is ok, the baby is fine. Call me later

"Come here, Anita, give me a hug. I think we both need one." Zara pulled her best friend close to her, hugging her tight. "Congratulations. You're going to be a mum."

"I know! I can't even describe how happy I am."

"You don't even have to. It's pretty clear from your teary eyes. Well, I suspect they are tears of happiness," Zara grinned.

Anita hugged her again.

"What are you up to now?" Zara asked, letting Anita go.

"Nothing much. I'm just going to shout into the world that I'm having a baby," Anita laughed.

"Good, and afterwards we'll go shopping to celebrate. I want to buy you something nice."

"Oh, ok. Thank you. Can I shout into the world while we are walking?"

"You can do whatever you want. You're now officially pregnant and can blame your behaviour on hormones."

"That's true. I'm a hormonal pregnant lady now. World, beware," Anita shrieked with a hint of evil, laughing wildly, and Zara joined in.

Both in an ecstatic mood, they were too happy to care about the surrounding people and what anyone thought of them.

Anita hunched up in the waiting room of the radiology centre. *This horrible nausea. Why did I book the scan for so early in the morning? God, how am I going to get through it?* she thought.

She glanced at George, sitting beside her, smiling. Beads of sweat popped out on her forehead.

I'm going to be sick. Where's the loo?

Anita frantically scanned the room for the toilet sign. She spotted the arrow in the corner and ran. *Oh no, it's coming. I'm not going to make it.* Dashing into the bathroom, she leaned over the toilet bowl and let it all out.

"Are you ok?" George asked with concern after Anita had returned to her seat.

"This morning sickness is the worst. I'm not ok yet, but should be fine soon. I usually vomit only until 10ish but the stupid nausea just hangs on. It never really goes away. I so can't wait for this to be over."

"When will it stop?"

"Soon, hopefully. Apparently, it's the worst for the first three months and I'm now at the end of those. It should be easing off now."

"Good. It must be tiring."

"It's more annoying than tiring; and mainly disgusting. I hate the taste of vomit in my mouth. It's so hard to get rid of," said Anita, popping a ginger sweet in her mouth. "Do you want one? They're supposed to help."

George laughed. "I don't have morning sickness."

"It doesn't matter. They're just sweets, you know? They're not specifically for pregnancy, so you could have one. I don't even know how many I have eaten in the last three weeks. I guess I'm supporting the whole company with this pregnancy."

"I'll still pass. I'm not that keen on ginger."

"Ms Wright?" the sonographer interrupted them. "Please, follow me."

Anita and George walked after the sonographer into a, to Anita familiar, room number 3.

Anita knew the drill already. She lowered her body onto the bed, unzipped her trousers, and lifted her top up. While doing so she thought, *this is the first time George is seeing a part of me naked. How odd that I'm not feeling embarrassed at all. Actually, why should I be? He doesn't like women in that sense, does he? It's not much different to me showing my stomach to Zara, is it?*

"This is your 12-week scan, Ms Wright. I will measure your baby and estimate your due date based on the actual measurements, rather than your last period. You will already be able to see the baby, and if interested, I can print some pictures for you."

"Yes please, we would love some pictures to show the family."

"Very well. Also, would you like the NT test done?" said the sonographer.

"What is the NT test?"

"It's a test to find out what the chances are of your baby having one of the known syndromes, including Down's. To do that, I would measure the baby's neck for nuchal translucency and later on, you would have a blood test. The collated information from these two would indicate the likelihood of your baby being affected."

Anita didn't want the test; she didn't care if the baby had one of these. Hell, she didn't care if the baby had two heads. Nothing would stop her from loving it, anyway.

"Would you like to discuss it in private?"

"No, we don't need to," said Anita. "I don't want the test. Just the normal scan, please."

George raised an eyebrow but said nothing.

"Ok then, we can start."

They watched the screen above, waiting for the sonographer to show them their baby. Anita gasped when a perfect human shape appeared on the screen. It was so different from the blurry images at 8 weeks. *There she is. There is my baby.*

George squeezed her hand, but Anita's eyes stayed glued to the screen.

My baby. She's perfect. She's absolutely beautiful. Just look at her. Anita's heart swelled with pride. *That's my own baby.*

"The baby looks well and happy. I'll take the measurements now."

The sonographer set to work while Anita admired the baby.

Oh, how her little legs move. She's already kicking. And her hands are waving around. She's such a wriggle. Oh my, she's so funny, look at her go.

The sonographer said, "I can't get clear measurements, because the baby is moving so much. It's extremely active for its age."

"Yes, it is, isn't it? It's jumping all over the place," said George.

"She's such a wriggle. It's so funny that I cannot feel anything. If she's almost doing somersaults, shouldn't I feel at least something?"

"No, not yet. The baby is still too little, and all the amniotic fluid is cushioning its movements. As the baby grows, you will feel it. But it needs to move less now, so I can take the measurements."

The sonographer kept on measuring the baby's size. "Ok, I have managed. I'll do the calculations now."

"This is the best telly ever," said Anita. "I could watch her forever."

"Based on the measurements," said the sonographer, "your baby is due September 6th, which is the same date calculated based on the day of your last period. The baby is right on time with growth."

"That's great, thank you. Can you print some pictures for us now?"

"Yes, I'll choose the best ones, where the baby is clearly visible." She chose six different images and printed them out.

"There will be a small charge for these," she said once she passed them the envelope.

"Of course."

"Well, that's it for today. We will see you again at your 20-week scan. Have a great day."

"We will, thank you. Bye."

Anita paid the bill and skipped outside into the chill of the wintery day. But not even the grey sky above dampened Anita's mood.

"Can I ask you a question?" said George. "Why didn't you want the NT scan?"

"Because I will love the baby whatever happens. If I knew the baby was likely to have the syndrome, it might persuade me to end the pregnancy, and I don't want to do that. I want her too much."

"Her. That's funny, you kept on saying her during the scan as well."

"Did I?" said Anita. "Oh, I guess I did. You're right! Well, for some reason, I think of her as a girl. Oh my, what if it's a boy?" Anita exclaimed. "Nah. I don't know why, but in my heart I know that the baby is a girl."

"We will have to wait and see, won't we?"

George grasped Anita's hand. "Thank you, Anita. You don't know how much being here with you today meant to me. Never in my wildest dreams I thought I would experience this. Seeing the baby kicking and rolling in your stomach was like ..., well, like magic. Thank you so much for allowing me to be here for this."

"You're welcome. It meant a lot to me that you came as well." Anita meant what she said. As much as she had tried to convince herself that she was more than happy to do this baby thing alone, she was grateful to have George by her side. It was beautiful to share this moment with him.

"Shall we split the pictures now? We've got six of them, so three and three is fair. And now, I am officially allowing you to tell your family. They'll be surprised, I imagine." Anita winked at George.

"Yes, pretty stunned, I expect. Telling them in person will be better, I suppose. Do you want to be there for it? My mum will think I'm pulling her leg otherwise."

"Well, I suppose I could. I'm free this coming weekend if you've got nothing on."

George lunged at her, hugging her. "Thank you so much." Seeing her startled expression, he pulled away. "I'm so sorry. I shouldn't have done that."

"That's ok, it just surprised me."

"Are you sure you will come with me?"

Anita nodded.

"It's a road trip then."

"Yes, it's a road trip. Just remember, I've got morning sickness and might need to spew," chuckled Anita. "But I'll try to do it into a bag."

"Well, I'd be grateful for that." George scrunched up his nose in a pretend disgust. "Otherwise, you will have to walk. They say pregnant women should exercise regularly, anyway. It will be good for you."

"Oh, so that's your secret plan, is it? How mean." But Anita's eyes betrayed her true feelings. Despite her nausea, she couldn't remember another time full of such pure joy. How glorious her life will be when the baby arrives.

"So, it looks like I'm going to meet George's family this weekend," said Anita to Zara, while talking on the phone the same evening.

"Are you?" said Zara in surprise. "That's ... good, I suppose."

Anita giggled, "Yes, exactly. I suppose it's good, but I don't know if I want to do it."

"Why are you going then?"

"Because I promised it. When we walked out of the clinic, George asked me to come with him. And, I was so happy and excited at that moment that I said yes, but now I'm having second thoughts and I don't really want to go. Oh Zara, how do I tell him I won't go? He'll be so upset."

"If you don't want to go, then don't. I don't think he'll be too upset. He'll understand."

"I'm not so sure. I know how important it is for him; he even hugged me when I said I would go."

"He didn't!"

"I know! You should have seen his startled face. He looked like a little boy who got caught stealing chocolate," giggled Anita.

"Poor George."

"Zara, I had never imagined meeting my donor's family. Never! And," Anita continued in a serious voice, "what if I'm still sick? I've been vomiting every morning; the nausea is not going away at all. I still feel as sick as I did two weeks ago. Apparently, it should ease off by the end of the first trimester. Not mine. Mine is still here in full force. What if I vomit throughout the car?"

"Well, what an introduction to his family," chuckled Zara. "Mum," she said, attempting to imitate George, "meet Anita, and please bring us a bucket of hot water and some cleaning rugs, because she spewed all over my car."

"Zara, it's not funny," said Anita, but even she had to laugh at the image. "Oh, it would be funny, wouldn't it? Afterwards, at least. I would be so embarrassed at that moment."

"Tell him you won't go because of the sickness."

"I might. I'll sleep on it and decide in the morning, but he's so excited. He's already messaged me to say he let his family know that he's coming this weekend and bringing a friend. And he's got a huge surprise for them. No pressure, right?"

"Anita, you don't owe him anything. As you said, this was never the plan. You have a contract signed, and this is not in it. You don't have any legal obligations to meet his family. Ever. So, don't let him pressure you into something you don't want to do."

"I know. And it's true, I don't have any legal obligations, but now we've become friends, things have changed. Maybe I should meet them so that I know who my child will be spending time with."

"Ok, just sleep on it and decide in the morning. But now, tell me about the baby of yours. I can't wait to see the pictures. You've got some, don't you?"

"Yes, yes, I've got printed scans to show you. She is beautiful, perfect already. The sonographer had problems measuring her because she was jumping all over the place. She's such a monkey already."

"Her? She? Did you already see the baby is a girl?"

"No, we didn't, but I know the baby is a girl, even though I'm not sure why. I just have this feeling inside me. So, if it's a boy, I'll be pretty surprised."

"Yes, I suppose you will. And you will probably be a bit disappointed too."

"I can never be disappointed with my baby, but in my heart I know that it's a girl. And if I'm wrong, I'm wrong. I won't care. It will still be my baby."

"No, you won't care, that's true."

"I'm having a baby, Zara. Half of the time, I still can't believe it. After all these years of trying, I have a baby in me. And you know what? As weird as it sounds, part of me is glad that I've been so sick."

"Really? Why?"

"Well, on the screen she was so wriggly, but I can't feel a thing, like nothing at all. You would expect that so much jumping would make me feel at least something, but the sonographer said the amniotic fluid is cushioning the activity for now. When she gets bigger, I'll start feeling her movements. But what I was saying, seeing how wriggly she is, I wouldn't know that I was pregnant if I wasn't sick. I would doubt it every second of the way. I cannot doubt it if I'm constantly nauseous, can I? Unless something is really wrong with me."

"That's true. Hopefully, the nausea stops soon though, so you can enjoy your pregnancy. They say you get that pregnancy glow at some point. I can't wait to see you shining," Zara laughed.

"Zara, you're being silly."

"Maybe, but it will be so much fun. When are you seeing the midwife?"

"In two weeks, and then the following appointments are going to be once a month, apparently."

"Good. Do you want to meet for lunch tomorrow so you can show me your baby?"

"What's tomorrow? Thursday? I can't. I've got only half an hour for lunch but we could have dinner together."

"Sounds great. Chris's got a meeting, anyway."

"Perfect. What shall we have?"

"Well, what can you have? You are so difficult at this moment," said Zara.

"It's not too bad. I'll bring something. My treat."

CHAPTER 19

"I'm so happy you're coming with me. Thanks again," said George after Anita had settled into his car on Saturday morning.

"No worries. We'll see how I survive it. I'm prepared for the worst," Anita smiled, showing George a collection of spew bags and ginger sweets.

"Is it still that horrible?"

"Yep, not getting any better. I'm still spewing until about 10 o'clock. So, we've got an interesting two-hour period in front of us."

"Oh good, so when we get to Mum's, you'll be better. The drive takes about two hours."

George looked pleased with the prospect. Anita didn't. She didn't want to throw up in front of him, and she will have to do it for two whole hours. Whoever said by the end of the first trimester things got better? Things were not better; if anything, they were worse. Anita was sick of being sick.

The morning sickness itself wouldn't be so bad if the nausea didn't last the whole day. She even suffered at night. When she spoke to Zara the night before, she had to run off to vomit. That hadn't happened often. Anita blamed it on both her morning sickness and the upcoming trip. She was quite nervous about meeting George's family. Zara's mouth dropped when Anita told her she had decided to go to Suffolk.

"Are you sure? It will be a weird meeting. Wouldn't it be better to do it later when you are well again?"

"I know and I'm expecting it to be odd, but I had promised it already. It wouldn't feel right to cancel it now. I'll be fine. I'll just have to be."

"Ok, your choice, but you'll have to tell me how they react to the news. Actually, just record it, will you? I would so love to see their faces."

"Zara, don't be silly. It won't be that bad."

"It won't be, you think? Their long-time gay son is bringing home a girl who he is having a child with. They will get the biggest shock of their lives."

Anita giggled, "You are right, it will be funny. I'm still nervous but actually looking forward to going now as well. What a surprise they'll get."

"Yep. So, be ready to recollect every second of it to me afterwards."

"I will. Don't worry a bit."

"How are you so far?" George interrupted Anita's pondering.

"Ok. Just drive smooth and don't go over any bumps. They make it worse."

"I'll try," said George. "I would rather not clean vomit out of my car."

"I'll aim well, I promise," said Anita, readying one of the spew bags.

They drove in silence for several minutes. Anita watched

the countryside passing by; the bleak English countryside with dry grass and bare trees. How she wished spring had already arrived. Winter made her suffering even worse. Sunny weather and new life popping out everywhere around would certainly lift her mood up.

They turned a corner and Anita's stomach flipped, her breakfast fighting its way into her throat. "STOP!" she shouted.

George pulled to the side of the road fast. Luckily, there were no cars behind them, otherwise his risky manoeuvre would have caused an accident. Anita flunked the door open and jumped out before the car even came to a full stop. Bending over a bush by the road, she vomited violently. Her stomach heaved again and again with more vomit covering the bare bush like Christmas tree ornaments.

"That's better," she said after returning to the car. "I shouldn't have eaten this morning. Now my whole breakfast is sitting in the bush." Anita drank some water and popped a ginger sweet in her mouth.

"Do you need more time, or shall I go?"

"You can go, I'm fine. It shouldn't come back for a while now."

How wrong Anita was.

"STOP!" she cried less than ten minutes later, jumping out of the car and, this time, decorating a clump of grass.

"I'm sure the baby's dancing a jig on my stomach," she sighed after returning. "Yes, that's what's happening for sure. That's why I'm still so sick. We saw how wild the baby was on the scan. She's just a monkey." Anita patted her stomach. "You stop dancing down there, will you? I'm barely surviving up here."

"Are you sure we should continue? Do you want to have a rest here or stop somewhere?"

George looked pale. Anita guessed he had only now grasped how bad she was.

"No, I want to go on. The sooner we get there, the better. I'll shut my eyes and try to snooze."

"Ok, as long as you're sure."

Anita closed her eyes, but no sleep came to her. George kept on glancing at her from time to time; she could hear his head turning. For once, she didn't mind the attention. It was quite nice to have someone caring about her.

The car went over a little hill, and Anita's stomach flew all the way up. There was no time to make it outside. She buried her head into the bag, emptying her stomach, while George shot her a worried glance.

"I'll stop now. A little rest area is coming up. We could both use some fresh air." George steered into the rest area and Anita clambered out of the car.

"I'm sorry, I know it smells," said Anita, throwing the bag into the rubbish bin by the single picnic table.

"No, you're fine. To tell you the truth, I'm surprised you are actually here. If I was this sick, I wouldn't be going on any trips. Why didn't you tell me how bad it was? I wouldn't be upset if you changed your mind and stayed at home. We could have gone at some other time."

"I did say I vomited every morning, but ... I didn't want to break the promise, and I hoped I would be feeling better already. I guess I'm not. We are not far away now, are we?"

"No, maybe another half hour or so," said George, checking his watch.

"Ok, I think I'll manage that; it should hopefully start settling now. I can't have anything left in me to spew, anyway." Anita walked to a little copse of trees at the edge of the rest stop and breathed deeply. The trip had gone as she had expected so far, so not very well at all.

"Take your time, Anita. We will continue when you're ready," George called after her.

"Thank you, I think I'm fine. The fresh air has helped. Let's go.

"Anita! We're here."

Anita woke up in shock.

"We are here." George pointed towards an old house with a large garden in front of it.

"Are we? I must have fallen asleep. Good."

Anita contemplated the white building with a thatched roof and large windows with dark green shutters. An arch spun above the entryway, with clipped rose bushes on both sides.

"Is this the house you grew up in? It's nice."

"Yes, this is where I was born. In this house. Mum had both of us here."

"Did she? How brave. I wouldn't be such a game."

Anita climbed out of the car, following George down the path towards the house. She noticed more rose bushes on both sides of the path and alongside the house and the fence line. Rose bushes surrounded the house like the castle in Sleeping Beauty.

"Your mum likes roses, doesn't she?"

"She loves them. You should see the house in summer when they are in full bloom. It's so beautiful that people come from far and wide to see it. They call it Rose Kingdom. But mum calls her house Rose Cottage." George pointed at the sign beside the door.

"Rose Cottage," Anita read aloud. "I would love to come again one summer. It must look amazing. And the smell. Oh my, the smell must be delightful."

The door opened, revealing a lady in her early seventies. "Oh dear! George, you are here already!" she exclaimed and hugged her son. "I expected you later. The roads must have been quiet."

"Yes, the drive was pretty easy; and we left early to beat the worst traffic."

George turned to Anita, "Mum, this is Anita. Anita Wright."

"Nice to meet you, Mrs Pearce," said Anita with her hand outstretched.

"Nice to meet you, Ms Wright."

George's mum shook Anita's hand with a curious expression. Her blue eyes darted from Anita to George and back, full of questions.

"Please call me Anita, Mrs Pearce."

"Oh, do come in, both of you," exclaimed George's mum, suddenly remembering that they were all still standing in the doorway.

George shot Anita an amused glance. Anita returned it. His poor mum looked so confused.

I'm sure I'm not the person she has been expecting. A new boyfriend, maybe, but certainly not a woman. But here I am, thought Anita.

Stepping into the house was like stepping into history. The house had obviously changed little in the last 50 years in both interior and exterior. The walls were lined with an old-fashioned wallpaper and the furniture had seen better days, but the house looked clean and tidy. Looking into the parlour, because that's what the first room on their left would be called, Anita was pretty sure the porcelain sets in the cupboards had never been used. Well, the entire room looked like that nobody ever went in.

This might change when a small child roams around here, chuckled Anita, *because judging by her wriggly nature, she will be unstoppable.*

George's mum led them into the kitchen. "I'll put some water on. Would you like a cup of tea, Ms Wright? I mean, Anita?"

"Yes please, I would love one."

Mrs Pearce went on, "I wasn't sure what the friend," she glanced at Anita, "George was bringing might like, so I made some scones and muffins, and I've got crisps and fruit as well. Help yourself to anything you like."

"Can I please use the loo?" asked Anita, feeling somewhat anxious about the upcoming conversation.

"Indeed, it's down the hall." Mrs Pearce pointed towards a door opposite to the front door, before continuing to organise things around the kitchen. Anita could see how much her hands shook. Her own anxiety getting the better of her, she excused herself and hurried away.

"So, what's happening? What is the surprise?" she heard the dreaded question being asked.

Anita dashed into the loo, not wanting to be part of it. She scowled at her reflection in the mirror. *I'm a complete mess. My hair is standing like I touched an electric fence, and is this a piece of vomit?* Anita picked something dry off her chin. *Yuck, what a great first impression I must have made. I should have checked my face in the car mirror first. Oh well, what's done is done.*

Washing her face with cold water and brushing her hair with wet hands, she stared in the mirror. *Hmm, not perfect, but much better.*

When Anita returned to the kitchen, George quickly swallowed his muffin and smiled. "And here she is. Mum can't wait to learn what our surprise is. I told her we would wait for you."

"You didn't have to. You could have shared the news without me."

"That wouldn't be fair, would it?"

I wouldn't mind at all, thought Anita, but she just smiled at George in response.

"Ok, you two, so tell me what the surprise is. Is it good? I hope it is good."

"You will want to sit down, Mum," suggested George. "It is quite big."

"Oh. Let me bring the cups to the table first." George's

mum sat the cups on the table, her hands shaking more than before, and scrambled for her own chair. "So, tell me; I'm ready."

"Well," said George, beaming at Anita, "you are going to be a grandmother."

"What? How? I mean, I know how. But you? Dear me." George's mum stared at them in disbelief.

"Yes, me, but it's not what you think. We are not a couple. I can't change who I am."

"Well, how did it come about, then?"

"Anita needed a donor, and I agreed. You know that I have always wanted a child, so we came to an agreement." He then set to explain about the contract and described what had happened since. He left out most of the personal bits, but still shared more than Anita felt comfortable with, and she found herself blushing at times. However, she let him take charge of the moment without joining in, content to just sit and listen.

"This is unusual, truly unusual," said George's mum finally after he had finished. "But joyful, of course, very joyful. Congratulations to both of you. Oh my, this is news I would have never expected from you," she grinned. "We need to tell your sister."

"Yes, we'll tell her tonight at dinner. They're coming, aren't they?"

"Yes, yes, they are. They should be here about five," said Mrs Pearce in a daze. "I still can't believe it. YOU are going to have a child. YOU!"

George grinned, excited at the prospect. "Yes, me."

"Finally alone," said Mrs Pearce after sending George to the shop to buy a few things for dinner.

Anita's heart jumped into her throat. *What did she mean*

by that? How I wish I had never come. Why did George have to leave me here?

"Now, I want to hear what is happening from you, Anita. It's been George talking all the time, like it doesn't concern you at all."

"Well, it does concern me, of course, but I didn't want to say much. You are George's family. It's his place to tell you, not mine."

"And what about your family? What are their thoughts on this um ... arrangement?"

Anita swallowed hard. "I don't have a family. My parents died in a car accident 11 years ago. I was the only child."

George's mum sat down. "I'm so sorry, my dear. It must have been hard for you."

"Thank you. It has been hard at times, I must admit. I'm extremely lucky to have a friend who has always been by my side. She is my rock; I don't know how I would have gone through the past years without her."

"That's good. I'm glad to hear you have someone like that in your life. Even though, and I'm just curious, that's all, but why did you want to have a baby like this? Why not meet a lovely young man and have a proper family? Aren't you worried the child will end up like you? With no actual family to speak of?"

Anita gasped. *How dare you question me like this?* she thought, but a brief shadow of doubt made its way into her mind. *She has a point, doesn't she? My baby will have nobody at all if something happens to me; she will be all alone. No, she won't, she will have George. She'll be ok. She'll be perfectly fine.*

Anita eyed George's mum, trying to figure out what she should say. *No need to turn this into an argument,* she decided. Instead, she replied, "I wanted a baby. Not a man. I don't like ... to be with men ... intimately."

Anita avoided George's mum's gaze; she was not

comfortable sharing her aversion, especially not with strangers, although this stranger will be her child's grandmother soon.

"Oh, I see," said Mrs Pearce. "Aren't there agencies or clinics that help people like you to get pregnant?"

"I've tried everything, trust me. I've tried to go the official way and I've tried to go the unofficial way, which almost cost me life." Mrs Pearce raised her eyebrows in question.

With the silent question hanging in the air, Anita's tap just opened, and she told her about her journey. The only two people who knew her entire story were Zara and her therapist. She needed to tell someone else, and George wasn't a woman. He wouldn't get it. So, she told George's mum about her applications and rejections; she told her about the trips to London. She told her about the miscarriages and the failed attempts with George. Once she started, she couldn't stop. All the details flew out. Every moment she regretted, all the pain she had suffered, every misfortune that had happened to her. And it felt good. No, it didn't feel good. It felt fantastic. When she had finished, she had tears streaming down her cheeks, but her soul and heart were flying right up in the sky. She felt lighter and relieved.

George's mum sat for good five minutes afterwards, processing what she had heard. At last, she walked over to Anita, who had regained some of her composure again.

"My poor girl, you've been through so much. You have had your share of bad luck, haven't you?"

She hugged Anita, who began to cry again.

"Things will be alright, you'll see. You're having your baby now, but I still need to ask you, what are your plans from now on? You've achieved your dream, so how does my son fit in it?"

Anita's insides bubbled as she stepped away from George's mother. *Has she not listened to anything?*

"What do you mean?" she hissed.

"I'm sorry, dear, I didn't want to anger you. I'm just trying to understand what will happen now. I don't want my son to end up hurt or penniless."

"Oh." Anita's temper still surging, she barked, "He will not. That's why we've got the legal agreement. I thought we had explained that enough. If nothing else, he will have the visiting rights specified in it, but because we have become friends since we had signed it, he will see the child more often. At least while we are on good terms. The agreement is going to stay in case something happens and we, for the lack of a better word, break up."

George's mum studied Anita without saying a word, so Anita spat, "Do you think I had planned on any of this happening? I didn't plan on meeting my donor's family. Ever. Especially not while I'm still pregnant. Maybe after the birth, during a special occasion in the child's life, but not like this. And, regarding George's um ... financial security," continued Anita, raging. "I can tell you in all honesty that I am not after his money. My parents had left me the house I live in and a nice sum of money I can live on. I wouldn't even have to work, but I do have a job. The only things George has to pay for are his personal trips with the child, as is written in the agreement. That's the only financial obligation he will be responsible for. I hope you're not expecting me to pay for his own personal costs."

Mrs Pearce said, "I'm sorry dear. I didn't mean to upset you. I had to make sure my son will be ok. You will understand my point once you have your own child. A mother will do anything for her child, anything. I like you and I can see George does, too. I'm glad you care for him as well and I'm thrilled to be a grandmother to your baby. Please excuse my questions. I just needed to know."

Anita's eyes filled with tears, her anger melting away. "I know you have concerns, but I promise that you have no reason to worry. We've considered all the aspects and issues that might arise."

George's mum grasped her hands. "I'm glad. I'm truly glad. Well, now," she let go of Anita's hands, "show me the pictures of my grandchild again."

"What happened here?" George's sight fell on Anita's teary face, his expression hardening.

"Nothing happened. Your mum and I had a nice little talk. That's all."

"A nice little upsetting talk, I see."

George turned to his mother. "Mum, what did you do? You know Anita is pregnant."

His mum raised her eyebrows. "Are you lecturing me on how to behave with a pregnant woman? When did you become a master at this topic? This is why I sent you to the shop. Otherwise, you wouldn't give me a chance to talk to this lovely girl on my own."

"George," said Anita, "you don't have to protect me. I can take care of myself."

George's eyes darted from one woman to the other. "I'm sorry," he said. "I think I have overreacted."

"You think? Maybe next time, you should think before you say something. Well, let me get this shopping sorted." She grabbed the bags, rolled her eyes, and started putting the food away. Anita heard her muttering something about men under her breath.

"Do you want to go for a walk, Anita?" said George. "It is nice around here."

"Yes, it will do me good."

"Are you sure you are fine? My mum can be intimidating," said George with concern once they were outside.

"I'm good, trust me." Then she added, "It was nice to talk to her. You're lucky to have a mother who cares for you so much. I would give anything for my mum to be here now." Anita's tears stung her eyes again. She swallowed hard to push them back.

"I'm sorry, Anita. I don't think I have been fully understanding what you are going through. It must be hard for you to do this without your parents. I need to start looking at things through your lens. First, I bring you here very sick and now this. I keep on missing your cues."

Anita sensed George's honesty. He meant what he had said. "It's fine, trust me. No harm done."

"Thank you. Let me show you around then. Down here is a nice little walk. You'll enjoy it, and then we could drive to town to look at the sights there, if you're still up for it. We should still have enough time before dinner."

"Shouldn't we help your mum with the dinner preparations?"

"Oh no, you won't be able to. Mum will send you away. She hates people in the kitchen. She says it all then takes her twice the time."

"Hmm, maybe she says that just to you. She might actually appreciate help from someone who can cook," Anita giggled.

"What? I can cook."

"Well, I have seen your shopping trolley, you know? And it was full of ready-made meals."

"That's just because I don't feel like cooking just for myself. I'll cook you a dinner next weekend, you'll see."

"Ok, I can't wait."

"Good; and then you can apologise," said George with a wink.

CHAPTER 20

"And this is your baby's head. You can see that all the features are well developed at 20 weeks already."

Anita watched the screen on the wall, George bobbing beside her with excitement.

"Do you want to know the sex of your baby?" asked the sonographer.

"No, we don't."

Anita had wanted to keep it a surprise. She didn't need to know. Zara was the complete opposite. She said she would want to get things ready, especially the nursery. Anita didn't mind at all. She had planned to use neutral colours and buy clothes both girls and boys could wear. Beige, green, yellow and cream were the colours of her choice.

"Ok, I'll tell you when to close your eyes or look away. I need to check the baby and you might recognise what the baby is even without me telling you," said the sonographer, continuing to move the probe across Anita's stomach.

"That's fine. Thank you," said Anita.

"First, I'll check the hands. Five fingers on each, moving well, no problems. Now the feet. Again, five toes on each. The baby is curled up in a nice little ball. Now, I will check the torso ... and the head. The baby looks well. I will move towards the intimate areas now, so please look away. If I can't see enough, I will ask you to walk around, hopefully turning the baby a bit."

Anita looked at George, who reluctantly turned his head away. She knew he didn't agree with her decision to keep the baby's sex a surprise. They discussed it, but Anita had the last word. When they visited George's family two months previously, the conversation steered in that direction, too. George's family were in unison, wanting to know if the baby was a girl or a boy, but Anita's mind was set. She loved surprises, and she wouldn't let anyone spoil the biggest surprise of her life. As long as the baby was healthy, actually, as long as the baby was here, her happiness was complete. The sex of the baby played no role.

"Ok, all done. I saw everything I needed. The baby is doing well. The growth and development are according to the age and all the organs and limbs are performing well. Your baby is healthy."

"Splendid. Thank you," said George. "Can we have some pictures?"

"Of course. Afterwards, please pay the charge at the front desk."

Anita and George walked out of the clinic, holding the precious pictures.

"How about we stop at the library and photocopy them? Then we can both keep the complete set," suggested Anita, studying the photos in detail. Each picture showed the baby from a different angle, and Anita wanted them all. "You could even photocopy them twice and send them to your mother as well."

"Great idea. She would love them; she's still so excited about this happening."

"You've got such a lovely family, George," admitted Anita. "I enjoyed my time in Suffolk. I worried so much before going, but they were all so welcoming. Especially your sister. She put me at ease almost instantly. Our situation is far from normal, but they accepted me with open arms and hearts."

"Thanks again for meeting them. It means so much to me. I know you didn't have to. The agreement states nothing like that, but you did, and I'm grateful."

Anita smiled at George. As much as she had been hesitant about meeting his family, Anita was glad she did. She knew now what background George had come from and saw in action how they all behaved towards each other. She saw all the love and respect among the members of his family and how happy his sister's children were. It filled her heart with joy. She knew that whenever her child wasn't with her, she would be loved. Or he would be loved, she had to remind herself. *But you are a girl, aren't you?* Anita stroked her stomach. *I know you are.*

"I can't believe you're halfway through your pregnancy already. You look so much better. Your vomiting has passed, hasn't it?" asked George.

"The time is flying, isn't it? 20 more weeks and we will get to meet our baby. I just can't wait," said Anita, smiling at the future prospect. "And yes, I'm better. I'm not well, but better. I stopped vomiting last week but I'm still nauseous, like the whole day. It's not as bad as before, but it's constantly here. I suppose I have learnt to live with it now, because sometimes I completely forget about it. But when I remember the baby, which is actually most of the time, nausea overcomes me so fast I have to take the ginger sweet. You know, those sweets have truly been life savers. I don't know what I would have done without them."

"You look so well; I would never have guessed you still had nausea. You are hiding it well."

"Good to know. It's part of my life now, I suppose."

"That's not fair."

"I'm ok, trust me, I would rather suffer knowing I'm having a baby than be well and still trying. This will be over soon."

What Anita didn't know was that unfortunately, the end to her suffering was nowhere near.

Anita walked to her midwife's office for her third appointment. She was supposed to have them once a month, but the busy clinic couldn't accommodate the schedule, so Anita's appointments were further apart than that.

"How are you, Anita?" her midwife, Debra, asked.

Anita didn't like this midwife, but with the huge midwife shortage, she had no other option; and she knew Debra didn't like her, either. At the beginning, Anita had to fill in a registration form. She wrote George's name and contact into the space for the father of the child. Further on, she ticked 'single' as her status. She knew Debra disapproved of this very much. The midwife made little remarks during their meetings to show her; remarks like: "Oh, these girls nowadays, getting pregnant before being married" or "A child needs a proper family, a father and a mother" or even better "I'm not sure what a girl is trying to prove when she gets pregnant without a man in her life". Debra tried to strip Anita off every piece of self-worth and downgraded her at every possible opportunity.

So, now when she had asked how she was, Anita reluctantly told her the truth. "I'm better. The vomiting has stopped, but I still feel nauseous pretty much the whole day."

"You can't be. That's impossible. You are over 24 weeks

already. All your morning sickness should have ended a long time ago. That can't be it."

Anita stared at her. She basically called her a liar and brushed off her symptoms as being only in her head. *I won't stress about this; I meet her only once a month. I will not complicate things,* Anita told herself.

"I've also been having sharp pains in my pelvic area. Well, not exactly in the pelvic area, it's more on the front. Like straight here." Anita pointed at her pubic bone.

"Having some aches and pains is a normal part of pregnancy. The baby is moving and growing, and so you must expect some strain on your body. The weight of the baby is pushing down and causing your pubic bone pain. That's normal. Don't worry about it."

"Well, is it likely to get worse?"

Debra cackled. "Yes, it is likely to get worse. As the baby gets bigger, the weight and the pressure on your body will also grow. Your pelvis needs to carry all the weight, and it needs to stretch to accommodate the growing baby. So, obviously, the pain in your pubic bone is likely to get worse. What a question."

Anita almost burst into tears. She could bear the pain if she knew she had the support she needed, but the tone of Debra's voice reminded her of the tone of her attacker. They both spoke with the same viciousness. The only difference being that Debra attacked her emotionally and all the scars were on the inside.

"Lie down on the bed and pull your top up, or even better, take it off. At least it won't keep on getting in my way like last time. I'll listen to the baby now."

As if in a trance, Anita obeyed the midwife's request. She just wanted to get through the appointment, go home and cry. The midwife didn't say, we will listen to the baby. No, Anita didn't matter.

A light knock on the door interrupted the examination.

"Come in," Debra called, not bothering about Anita's half naked body. This woman undeniably didn't care about her at all.

A young woman with dark red hair entered. "Hi Debra, I'm here to meet Ms Wright. Is this a good time?" she smiled at Anita.

"Well, you're already here, so you might as well stay," Debra barked. "This is Anita Wright. Anita, this is one of my colleagues, Josie Bell. She'll be your backup midwife; in case I'm busy at a birth or something more important has come up."

The way she said it made Anita understand that everything and anything in the world was more important than her and her baby.

Anita pulled up to meet the new midwife.

"No, please, stay lying down. Nice to meet you, Ms Wright. May I call you Anita?"

"Absolutely."

Anita liked this girl; she was so much nicer and caring than Debra. Why, oh why, couldn't this be her main midwife?

"Ok, you've met her. Now give us a chance to finish this appointment," said Debra.

"Of course. I'm sorry I have interrupted. Nice to meet you, Anita."

Anita smiled at Josie as she was leaving. Knowing there were kind midwives, but she had this horrible woman almost made her cry. However, she knew she would give this woman another reason to despise her if she burst into tears, a reason to degrade her even more. Instead, she put a brave face on and finished her appointment.

Once at home, all the suppressed emotions exploded and Anita cried and cried until she had no tears left. And after that, she sobbed tearless sobs, her body heaving.

CHAPTER 21

"What you are experiencing can't be normal, Anita," said Zara, sitting in Anita's kitchen with a cup of tea in her hand. "You don't see other pregnant women walking around in so much pain."

"That's exactly what I messaged to the stupid midwife. I even cannot sit on the chair; it hurts so much. All she said was to get myself a pregnancy belt because what I'm experiencing is part of being pregnant. She just doesn't like me. Not at all."

"Well, at least it's mutual," laughed Zara.

"Yes, it for sure is. I wish I had the other woman, the back-up midwife. She seemed so nice."

"When is your next appointment?"

"In two weeks. I'm only 27 weeks now. When the baby gets bigger, how will I move?"

"So, when does it hurt the most?"

Anita shifted uneasily on the chair. She had a cushion

underneath her to try to soften the impact, but her pubic bone still hurt. It had been giving her such grief in the last few weeks, hurting more and more each day.

"When I'm sitting, as you can see, and when I'm getting up from a sitting or lying position. That's a complete nightmare. Walking up and down the stairs and standing for a longer period is excruciating. It's better once I get going. Sometimes it even almost stops. I guess it freezes up when I don't move for a while." Anita leaned back in her chair, relieving the pressure on her pubic bone. "The worst is when I need to go toilet in the middle of the night because I can't get up. It takes me such a long time to start moving and I have to hold the walls for support to actually make it to the loo at all."

Zara looked at her friend with concern. "You haven't got the pregnancy belt yet, have you?"

"No, I need to order something online. I don't know of a shop in Maidenhead where you can buy them, and I don't want to go trampling around the shops in this state."

"Oh, there's a little maternity shop, just off High Street," said Zara. "They should have them."

"How do you know? I don't know that there's a shop like that and I'm pregnant, not you."

"I ...," began Zara, "came across it by an accident the other day."

Anita stared at Zara. Something felt odd about the way she said it. "Did you? By an accident? Zara, what's going on."

"Well, umm ..., I might have had a positive test."

"Seriously? Are you pregnant?"

"I think so."

"And when were you going to tell me?"

"Today. The perfect moment hasn't come yet. I didn't want to steal your storm, especially now when you are this sore."

"Oh Zara, this is the best news. Come and give me a hug."

Zara jumped up and hugged Anita tight.

"Congratulations."

"Thank you."

"Were you trying?" Anita asked when Zara had sat down again.

"No, we were not. We still wanted to wait, but you know how my periods are. I can never rely on them."

"But you are happy, aren't you?"

"Oh yes, ecstatic. And Chris is so excited. It's pretty cute, if you ask me."

"So, when are you due? It must be about half a year after me."

"Yes, pretty much," said Zara. "With my periods being so irregular, the date is still unconfirmed. They will tell me at the dating scan. But it's likely to be around the beginning of March. The dating scan is not until week 12, though. How did you ever wait this long? I want the scan right now," Zara moaned.

"It will be here before you know it. Don't worry. I hope your morning sickness won't be as bad as mine. I wouldn't wish that on my worst enemy. Well, maybe on the stupid midwife." Anita sneered at the thought of Debra spewing violently.

"Has it gone now? You've got enough problems with your pelvis as it is."

"You know what? Yes, it has gone. Since the pain in my pelvis got worse, I stopped feeling sick. Maybe it is like the midwife said and it was all in my head. Who knows?"

"Yeah, nah, that won't be it. It's more likely that you finally passed the sickness period. Or, you know how sometimes when something hurts you but something worse happens and hurts more, then the first pain disappears? You're not crazy, Anita." Zara grinned with a cheeky expression. "I mean, you are crazy. Look what you have put your body through, but you are not crazy enough to make yourself feel sick."

"Thank you, Zara. It's nice to know that you think I'm crazy," Anita laughed.

This is what she needed, an honest conversation with Zara. She had always made things better, no matter what the problem.

"Shall we pop into the maternity shop? Are you up for it?" Zara winked at Anita. "I can pull and push you if needed."

"I should manage, but thank you for the offer. Maybe, in a few weeks' time, I'll take you up on it," said Anita. "Here I go!"

Holding onto the table, she got up. Sharp, piercing pain, as if somebody jabbed a long needle into her body, shot through her pubic bone. She made the first few hard steps before the pain begun to ease. By the time she walked to the door, the pain subsided.

"See? I'll be ok. I just can't stay in one position for too long."

"Good, I'll be running you around the block, then. If it helps, I'm happy to do that for you. That's the sacrifice I'm ready to make."

Anita giggled. "You always know how to pick me up. Let's go then. Come and shove me into the car."

"At your service, my queen."

Anita stared at her reflection in the mirror. She smirked at the ridiculous look. The lady at the shop recommended her a pregnancy belt, which had an additional strap for the top of her bump. Apparently, it provided more comfort than just the bottom strap ones. It might have provided more comfort, not that Anita had anything to compare it with, but her bump looked like in prison; only the tip of her belly with her protruding bellybutton showing.

Oh well, if it helps, I'll wear it. I can imagine how boiling I will be in the summer when the heat hits, she grunted.

English weather was generally mild, but the weather forecasters were promising a scorching summer that year. Anita turned this way and that, confirming the side view was as bad as the front one. *It will be all underneath my clothes anyway, so who cares?*

At night, Anita had to go to the loo. She turned onto her right side, trying to get up, the pain in her pubic bone unbearable. She sat up, huffing, "For goodness' sake, how bad will this still get?" Stumbling to her feet and holding the wall, she limped to the bathroom. When she finally lowered her body onto the toilet seat, she burst into tears. "I need help. I can't go on like this."

Sleep was out of the question. Instead, Anita turned her computer on to research the pain she had been suffering from. It didn't take her long to locate articles on pelvic girdle pain and symphysis pubis dysfunction. Most of the described symptoms fitted her pain. Anita read lots of advice on dealing with the pain, practical solutions worth trying. The recommendations ranged from walking up and down the stairs sideways, not crossing legs, sleeping on the side with a cushion in between legs, to not pushing or lifting anything heavy. Vacuuming and standing on one leg were also not advised. *Oh good, I have an excuse not to vacuum,* Anita snorted.

Knowing what her issue might be brought at least some clarity into her mind. None of the articles mentioned a pregnancy belt as a solution. *Yes, because the stupid midwife doesn't want to deal with me.*

However, Anita had decided to mention this to her and ask for a referral to a specialist.

"You are perfectly well. No need to bother a specialist. What you are experiencing is not SPD. Women with SPD can barely walk, but you walked in here just fine."

Debra wouldn't hear a bar of Anita's complaints. She still ignored her pain.

"But I didn't walk in here just fine. I had to go up the steps sideways, and I walked to the clinic rather than take the car because I wouldn't be able to get out of it. I am not ok and you telling me I am is making me livid. You don't have to cope with the pain I'm experiencing, and I request you to write me a referral to a specialist," exclaimed Anita, raising her voice and letting all the frustration she had been feeling with this woman out.

"How dare you talk to me like this? You got yourself into this so you can suffer for it. I'm not writing you a referral. You bear the consequences of your actions."

"Pardon me? You don't even know how I got pregnant. You just saw that I was single and judge me based on that. You are such a bitter old woman and I don't want you to be my midwife anymore. I'm going to complain and request someone else."

Debra snickered, "And you expect midwives are queuing to take you on, do you? You expect we have anyone available so close to your birth? You're clueless. We are so swamped with women it's not funny. Like it or not, you are stuck with me."

"No, I'm not. I don't want you to be birthing my child. I would rather give birth on my own than have you there. Goodbye." Anita heaved her body up. Shaking with anger, but bursting with pride, she limped out of the room. She didn't like conflict, and she had never defended her rights in such a way. But she had to now. She was suffering, and the hag didn't care at all.

Anita waddled to the reception desk.

"May I help you?" the receptionist asked.

"Yes. My name is Anita Wright, and I would like to change my midwife."

"I'm not sure if we can do that. All our midwives are full. Who is your current midwife, and why do you want to change?"

"Debra Lawson. She has been the most unsupportive person since the beginning. She doesn't care about my pain and brushes it off as a normal pregnancy niggle. I cannot walk and move and she won't write me a referral to a specialist; and she keeps on putting me down, harassing really, because I'm single. I'll be laying a formal complaint to the Midwifery Council."

"Oh, ok, I'll see what I can do. Do you know who your back up midwife is?"

"Josie Bell."

The young woman typed something into the computer, gazing at the screen. She pursed her lips as she worked, trying to find a solution.

"You are not helping this woman, are you?" an angry voice boomed behind Anita. She turned to face Debra Lawson. "She is my client and you are not moving her to anyone else."

"I have the right to refuse your services, and that's what I'm doing. You are not my midwife anymore."

Debra turned to the young woman, "You will not give her an alternative midwife, or else ..." She let the sentence hang. The young woman's eyes flashed with fear and her whole composure changed, with her body slumping further behind her desk.

Anita's blood boiled. She wasn't this woman's puppet and the receptionist neither.

"You cannot talk to this lady like this. You don't have the right. And you don't have the right to keep me as your client.

I'm going to write a formal complaint to the Council, your behaviour is awful and absolutely unacceptable. You are such a bully."

Debra turned white and hissed, "And what do you think the Council will do? I have a clean record and with the shortage of midwives, they'll do nothing. You're wasting your time and efforts."

"Maybe, but I will not know until I try, will I?"

Debra gave her a look that could kill, turned on her heel and stormed out of the area.

The receptionist groaned. "She's going to make my life hell now."

"If she tries anything, contact me. I'm going to write into the complaint that she threatened you as well. We cannot let her bully you, or me, or any other woman who works or comes here."

"But she's correct, you know? The shortage is real and the Council won't do anything about it."

"They might and they might not. I will still complain. Now, can you please check if you have anyone else available? Otherwise, I'll need to search for a private midwife, which I should have done straight at the beginning, but I figured a public one would be ok. And now all of them will be full for my due date," Anita despaired. "What happens if I don't have a midwife?"

"Hold on, Josie might actually have one spot left. Let me confirm with her."

Anita held all of her fingers and toes crossed while the receptionist called Josie.

"Hi Josie, here is Janet. I've got a young woman, Anita Wright, here. She is one of Debra's clients."

Anita was glad to learn the woman's name; their relationship seemed much more personal now. She watched her listening to Josie on the other end, her patience dwindling.

"Oh, you have met her, have you? Good. Well, Ms Wright had a ... rife with Debra and is requesting a change in midwife. Any chance you could take her on? She's due September 6th."

Janet listened. "Yes, she is here with me. I can pass her the phone if you'd like."

Janet gave Anita the receiver. "Josie would like to talk to you."

"Hello, here is Anita."

"Hello Anita. I understand you and Debra have had a bit of a misunderstanding."

"Yes, I have. Debra has been downgrading my symptoms since the beginning and today wouldn't write me a referral to a specialist because I suspect I have SPD. I can barely move but she says I'm ok and don't need anything. According to her, all my pain is a normal part of being pregnant. It sounds petty, but she is also so rude and doesn't respect my decision to have a baby as a single woman. I can't cooperate with a bully. She threatened Janet here as well if she tried to help me."

"She did? I'm sorry. I can take you on if you'd like, but we won't be able to have an appointment until the end of next week. Will that work for you?"

"Yes, definitely. Thank you."

"In the meantime, I can email you a referral to a physiotherapist if you'd like. However, do you know that you can book yourself to see a private specialist? You don't need a referral from anyone. And, to be honest, I would recommend you do just that. You could wait for a public health system physiotherapist for a few weeks or even months. They tend to get very busy. The private one will be more expensive, but if you are in so much pain and can afford it, the sooner you deal with it, the better."

"I can? I didn't know that. Why didn't Debra tell me that? I will definitely look some up. Thank you so much."

"No need to thank me. I don't want you to be in pain. Some pain is normal in pregnancy, but SPD is not. Even if you don't have it, a physiotherapist will advise how to deal with the pain you have. Who might actually be even better is an osteopath. They work with the whole body and the results for this sort of pain can be better. You could try both of them."

Anita's eyes welled with tears at the different treatment. "Thank you, thank you so much."

"You're welcome. I'll email you the referral straight away if you'd rather go with a public one, and I'll see you next Friday at 2pm. Does the time suit?"

"Yes, perfect. Thank you again."

Anita gave the phone back to Janet. "She will take me on. Thank you for your help."

"I'm happy for you. All women deserve to have a good pregnancy experience."

"I agree. Well, I'll get out of your hair now. If anything happens with Debra, please contact me. I'm going to write the complaint letter still today."

"I will. Thanks."

Anita hobbled outside a changed woman. She was so pleased with the result she had achieved. If she could dance, she would.

CHAPTER 22

"The symptoms you are describing suggest pelvic girdle pain. When did you say the pain started?"

Anita perched on the edge of the chair at the osteopath's practice. The clinic had a cancellation, and she was able to schedule an appointment for the very next day. She didn't want to wait weeks for a public specialist and she had the money to cover the bills, so it made total sense. She had lost enough time already thanks to that horrible woman and lived with the pain for too long.

"It started at about 24 weeks, now I'm 29."

Lauren, the osteopath, blinked her eyes in surprise. "You have been in all this pain for five weeks already? You should have come earlier. We could have dealt with it and made you more comfortable."

Anita teared up. "I would have if I knew that I could book a private appointment on my own. I told the midwife several times how sore I was and asked her for a referral, but she kept on refusing, saying that I didn't need it. I can't get out of bed at night and walk, but it is apparently not bad enough to 'bother a specialist'. These are her exact words."

"Well, you can take my report to your midwife, because based on what you said, it is pretty bad."

"Thank you for acknowledging it. I have doubted my sanity already. She is not my midwife anymore. I have requested a change."

"Good on you. Well, we need to do a proper examination now. Can you lie down on the bed? I'm afraid some positions and movements I'll perform will be probably uncomfortable. I need to look at your body, especially joints, and how they move and establish the level of pain you are in."

"That's ok. Do what you have to do. I'm ready to do anything to relieve the pain I'm in."

Anita struggled up, her pelvis stiff and pubic bone sore. She made the few steps to the bed and sat down heavily.

"Did this hurt you?" asked Lauren, who noticed Anita's issues.

"Yes, it always hurts more when I stay in one position for a longer period. Especially chairs are not my friends at the moment with my pubic bone hurting a lot while I'm sitting down. I have to sit on the edge of the chair for it to feel at least a bit better. I guess the pressure is then on a different area, but I don't really know. I have been using a yoga ball at home. It makes some difference, but after a while, it still starts hurting even on it."

"I see. Well, can you lie on your back, please?"

Anita lowered her body onto the bed.

"I will examine you now. Let me know if the pain gets worse while I move your limbs."

Lauren picked up one of Anita's legs and moved it upward and sideways. Anita hissed in pain.

"This was sore, wasn't it?"

Anita nodded.

"I'll try your other leg now."

Yet again, Anita hissed in pain.

"I'm sorry. Can you move onto your side now, please?"

The osteopath did similar movements with Anita's legs while she was lying first on one and then on the other side. Afterwards, she examined her torso and pelvic area in a standing position. Some movements brought on more pain and some didn't hurt at all.

"You seem to be suffering from a high level of pain, Ms Wright. I wish I have seen you earlier."

Anita's face must have shown her dismay.

"It's ok, I can still help you. However, you'll need more sessions. The treatment will take longer than if you had come earlier, unfortunately."

"What a relief that you can still help me. Thank you. I can't go on like this until the birth."

"No, you can't. And not always the pain stops after giving birth, either. You could still suffer from it afterwards, on a certain level. I'll do some exercises to help you now. Can you lie back on the bed? I will move your body in specific ways that should shift your bones, ligaments and muscles and relieve the pain, eventually. We will do similar treatment while you are standing up."

Anita spent about an hour at the osteopath's that day. Some exercises were uncomfortable, and some even brought tears into her eyes. She only hoped they would be worth it in the end. Lauren gave her an exercise to do at home several times a day, too. Anita had to sit on a low chair, with her legs bent at a right angle and her back straight. She had to close her legs together while pushing against them with the palms of her hands. The applied pressure was meant to release the muscles and bones around the pelvic area. It sounded like a weird exercise, but Anita had to trust the specialist. She had nothing else left.

"I feel like I'm living at the doctors now," said Anita when she met with Zara the following weekend.

"Is it helping, though?"

"It is. I'm still in pain, but I can walk now. I've had two sessions already and one more booked for next week. The osteo said I might need two more, but the next two can be two or three weeks apart. She's thrilled with the progress we have made. And so am I, naturally."

"Brilliant. I'm so happy for you. Living in constant pain must be awful."

"And how are you Zara? Any morning sickness?"

At five weeks pregnant, Anita already vomited every morning.

"Well, I have been nauseous in the mornings, but haven't spewed once. I hope it won't come at all; I don't like vomiting." Zara made a disgusted face.

Anita laughed, "Who would like it? I hope you don't get much of it. It wasn't fun."

"So, how's the new midwife? You had your first appointment with her, didn't you?"

"She's amazing, so kind and caring. She showed so much concern for me and my troubles. I confided in her about the way I got pregnant. I would have never dreamed of telling the other one. And you know what? She congratulated me on finding a way. I'm so happy I had requested the change. So happy."

"I can imagine, hun. What about the complaint? Any news?"

Anita wrote the letter of complaint the day after the incident and emailed it to the Midwifery Council.

"I haven't had anything back yet. The initial response said that it could take several weeks to investigate. So, I'm not sure when and if I'll get anything back."

"At least you complained. The woman deserved it for sure."

"She did. What a hag. I can't believe such a woman can be a midwife. She has no people skills and no idea how to talk to expectant mothers who are hormonal already. She is a bully, that's what she is. I caught up with the receptionist, Janet, yesterday. I am worried about her. She still needs to be in the same building, but she said that Debra hadn't bothered her at all. Apparently, she walks past her without even acknowledging her presence."

"You can't please some people," said Zara. "My first midwife appointment is soon; her name is Gabrielle. Hopefully she's more like your Josie than Debra. After your experience, I'm so anxious to meet her."

"I'm sure she will be lovely. It's impossible for two midwives to be like Debra. She's one of a kind." Anita grasped her friend's hand. "You will have the best pregnancy ever. I know it."

"Anita, I hope you're correct. I so wish you haven't been through all of this. It's not fair for one person to suffer this much."

"I'm ok, Zara. I promise. I'm doing fine. And you know what? Because I've been having all these issues, my birth is going to be quick. I just know it."

"I'm sure it will. Speaking of birth, are you still planning to do the hypnobirthing classes? I've read up on it and it sounds interesting."

"I am. I'm booked into them already. The first class is next week. Apparently, I should have started earlier because the longer you do it, the better results you gain out of them, but, oh well, it can't be helped now, can it?"

"Oh, so you can go to the lessons earlier. Could I start like now?"

Anita grinned at her friend in excitement. "Yes, we can do it together. How awesome will that be? My class is on

Tuesday evenings at 7. See if they still have a space then. If not, the other class is on Thursdays and maybe I could rebook into that one."

"Sounds like a plan. I'll get onto it today. Can I book online?"

"Yes, yes," confirmed Anita. "I did the booking online. Oh, this is perfect. I'm looking forward to it even more now."

"How did you like the class?" Zara asked Anita when they walked out of the community centre after their first hypnobirthing lesson.

"I loved it," said Anita. "I thought it was really good. I'm so relaxed and actually looking forward to the birth. How funny is that? And that's only after one lesson. How am I going to feel after I've done five or six?"

"I agree. Parts of the class were more like meditation than anything."

"Yes, they were. I hope I'll be able to get my mind into the 'uplifting state allowing my body to perform to its best ability'," said Anita, mimicking Theresa, the hypnobirthing teacher. "Apparently, the body knows what to do. Well, we'll see. My body has betrayed me before more than once."

"Yes, but you sorted it out and now it will listen to you."

"I hope you're right. This dream has brought a lot of pain to me already."

"I just wish I knew Chris should have come, too. All those couples attending and the two of us together. Did you see them looking at us? We were like animals at the Zoo," Zara chuckled. "I would have expected more of an open mind from people nowadays. Oh well, it doesn't matter. He can come next time."

"Oh yes, sorry, that was my fault. When I spoke to Theresa before signing up, I didn't even ask her about a partner. George won't be coming to the birth, so to me it didn't matter."

"No worries, I should have enquired myself. How are you and George, by the way? You haven't spoken about him for a while and I haven't asked either. So much has been happening now."

Anita smiled, "Yes, the beginning of pregnancy was busy for me, too. Not because I had a lot to do, rather I had no time for anyone or anything else. I get where you're coming from."

"It's weird, isn't it? I had so much time before and now it's all gone. And I don't know where. So, what about George?"

"George is good," Anita said while walking to the car. "He contacts me pretty much every day, sometimes only with a quick message, but most of the time, he calls. And from time to time, we catch up for a cup of tea. He's been supportive and helpful. He's definitely looking forward to the baby."

"Are you sure you don't want him to be at the birth? Wouldn't it be nice to have him by your side when the baby comes?"

Anita looked at Zara in alarm. "No! I can't imagine him standing beside me when I'm pushing the child out, with all my private parts exposed to the world. He's not like Chris, who has seen everything you have to show Zara. George is supposed to be just a donor, nothing else. He wasn't supposed to be involved this much in my life as it is."

"True, he wasn't," said Zara, unlocking the car.

Anita stopped, "Oh Zara, I hope I'm not wrong in letting him to be this involved. It still feels, umm, odd. I have never planned for this to happen. This is my baby, and I don't know if I'll be able to share her with George as much as I'll have to."

"Anita, it will be fine. It will take some time to adjust to the fact the baby has a real father, that's true, but George will not be taking the baby away until she's older. Isn't that what you agreed on?"

"True. It's not until the child is older. I think he can't imagine dealing with a baby on his own."

"And can you?"

"Can I what?"

"Well, can you imagine dealing with a baby on your own?"

"I'm a bit scared, naturally. The children at my nursery are all older and I've never had to look after a tiny newborn, but that's what most first-time mothers go through, isn't it? They don't have the experience the first time around and I'm pretty confident I'll manage. I'll have to. What else can I do?"

"Give her to George!" laughed Zara, keeping her eyes on the traffic. "See? Isn't it great to have a back-up plan for when you get overwhelmed? You'll be able to call on George to come and help."

"True, I will. It will be a good thing to have him around, won't it? He can take her for walks during the day and I can have a nap. Oh yes, I like this plan," said Anita, bobbing up and down.

"I'm glad you're so happy. You're obviously in much less pain than the last time I saw you."

"Yep, my body is getting back to normal now, at least during the day. The nights are still bad and the wall is my best friend. I should have invested into an old people walker," Anita chuckled.

"I wish the horrid midwife told you to book a private osteo straight away."

"Yeah, I suspect she liked to see me suffer. Otherwise, why would she do it?"

"I hope they'll kick her butt off the midwife registry. She's a disgrace to the profession."

"I don't want to talk about that bully; it still makes me upset," said Anita.

"Umm, what do you think about the placenta encapsulation?" asked Anita instead.

"You mean eating my own placenta after giving birth? Yuck, that sounds disgusting. I don't know how anyone can do it. And why?"

"It's supposed to be good for your body and for the baby, too. It gives your body back the nutrients you lost because of having the baby, so that you recover faster."

"Yes, Theresa said that, but I'm still not convinced it's true. I would feel like a cannibal eating my own insides." Zara pretended to gag. "Yuck."

"Well," Anita said, "I might do it."

Zara stared at her, almost swerving into the opposite lane. "You must be joking."

"I mean, I want to do more research on it, but I like the idea. It sounds beneficial."

"But it's not normal to eat your insides, Anita!"

Anita considered what Zara had said for a moment. She could see her friend didn't agree with the idea, and whatever Anita said wouldn't change her mind.

"My journey to this point hasn't been normal, Zara, you must admit that. I actually don't find it disgusting. It will be in capsules, so like eating vitamins anyway. I won't be able to taste it."

"You do you, Anita, and I'll do me. No way you'll talk me into doing it. My stomach turns upside down just listening to you."

"Anyway, here we are. I have to go straight home; Grandpa's got an early appointment tomorrow, so I need to get some sleep."

"No worries. Good night, Zara. We'll talk soon," said Anita, scrambling out of the car, hoping her friend wasn't upset about the placenta discussion.

She unlocked and opened her front door, waved to Zara, and walked in.

Anita was exhausted, the baby eating up all her energy.

"You're tiring me out, little one. How about we try to sleep now? And no kicking tonight, alright?" said Anita, rubbing her belly while walking upstairs to her bedroom.

CHAPTER 23

"And my pain is almost gone now," Anita summed up her osteo treatments to Josie, her new midwife.

"That's great. I'm so happy to hear that. Some pain in pregnancy is inevitable, of course. You've got a baby growing in you and it is pushing on your organs. Your body is stretching in ways you would have never deemed possible and your bones are shifting, too. Pregnancy puts a lot of strain on the body, so it's not surprising you hurt, but if we can find means to relieve the pain, and help you to learn to manage it, these ways need to be explored," said Josie, making some notes into Anita's file.

"Thank you again for taking me on. Debra and I clashed so much, and I would have still been suffering under her care."

"We each have our own methods," said Josie. "And we each use a different approach."

"Well, I like your approach much better," smiled Anita.

"You know what's funny? From all I've read, the third trimester is supposed to be the worst. For me, it will actually be the best. The first two trimesters were a complete write off, and I didn't enjoy them at all, but now I'm feeling great. I'm almost pain free, the baby is moving around and kicking, and I'm so happy."

Josie smiled back at her. "That's wonderful, Anita. Ok, we need to write your birth plan now. I see you haven't done one yet."

"What do you mean by a birth plan?" Anita asked in confusion.

"We will write down how you would like your birth to go, what you want to happen once your time comes. It's better to have it written now because you won't be thinking clearly when it is happening."

"Oh, ok, I see."

Josie looked at her notes. "First, we need to establish your birthing place."

"Do I have options?"

"You do. The most typical is in the hospital, but you can also choose a birthing centre, or even birth at home."

"Well, ... I guess I'll go to the hospital, that seems like the safest option. If something goes wrong, I would like to have doctors who can help nearby."

"Very well. Now, how do you want your birth to progress? Do you want to use gas or air, or any other medication, or even epidural?"

"I want my birth to be as natural as possible. So, no epidural or other medication unless it can't be avoided, only air please. I have also joined hypnobirthing classes this week."

"Have you? That's good. I have heard great things about hypnobirthing, although none of my clients has ever done it, so I don't have any experience in it. Ok, I will write that you only prefer air."

"What about water birth?"

"Oh, yes please, I've read a lot about water birth and it seems easier. Is it?" Anita asked in a hopeful tone.

"In general, it can be. Water helps your body to relax and soothes it while you're in labour. The baby also exits from water to water, so it's not such a shock either; entering the world must be a stressful experience for an infant. Well, that's my opinion, anyway," Josie said.

"Yes, I would like a water birth. It sounds peaceful."

"Great, and who are you going to have at birth?"

"Umm, no one, just me. I hope it's not an issue."

"No, of course not. I only need to know how many extra people will be in the room."

"Oh, ok. Only me in the room. The father will wait outside and my friend Zara as well."

"Good. We also need to discuss cord clamping. We can cut the cord straight after the baby is born or wait. I personally recommend delayed clamping. My preferred method is, once the baby is born, we lay the newborn on the mother. Skin to skin contact is vital as it means that you will begin your bonding process straight away, and the baby will want to feed. Some infants are quick. It is amazing how they naturally attach to the breast, seeking milk. They can smell it, you know?"

Anita read a lot of articles about birth and was thrilled this midwife wanted the same birth she had dreamed of.

"After a while, we clamp the cord," Josie continued. "After birth, the cord is still full of nutrients, and delaying the clamping allows them to pass to the baby. Is that what you want to do?"

"Yes, please delay the clamping. That sounds much better."

"Perfect. Now, what about the vitamin K injection for the baby? Do you want your baby to have it? If you choose to, it has to be injected straight after birth or the baby can take several oral doses afterwards. The injection is a preferred method, however."

"What is it for?" asked Anita.

"For a disorder called haemorrhagic disease, which can happen in newborn babies. This disease causes bleeding and Vitamin K helps to prevent this. It is a rare disorder but, if not treated in time, can cause permanent issues and sometimes be fatal."

"And the injection is safe, is it? Do you recommend it personally or because it is normally done?" The idea of her newborn being injected straight away scared Anita.

"I do recommend it personally. It is not worth the risk."

Anita sat thinking for a while. "Ok, let's do it."

"Great."

"And for you, I will offer you an injection of oxytocin after birth. This will stimulate contractions and your body will push the placenta out more efficiently. Your choice to have it or not."

"Well, speaking of placenta. I want to have my placenta encapsulated. Can this injection harm the placenta in any way? I mean, does the drug in the injection have time to enter the placenta?"

"Without the injection, placenta delivery can take up to an hour, with it about half an hour. In my opinion, the oxytocin might have time to enter your placenta, but I can't tell you if and how it might affect it. You need to do some more research on it yourself."

"Thank you for being honest with me. I'll stay away from the oxytocin injection to start with and if it looks like the placenta is not coming, I'll reconsider," said Anita. "Is that an option?"

"This is your birth and your body; you decide what happens. Have you booked a service for the encapsulation?"

"No, I haven't. The lady running the hypnobirthing classes had recommended it and had given us two contacts.

I'm going to call them today to check if either of them is available for my due date. I wasn't sure about it until today, but the more I read on it, the more I want to do it. It will be good for me. It will be good for us."

"Yes, it can be helpful because the placenta is full of nutrients. I suppose little research has been done on the topic to fully establish the benefits. Some people eat placenta raw or cooked, some people freeze it, some plant it in their garden, and some people leave their placenta at the hospital, not wanting to deal with it. It's every mother's choice to do as she wishes."

"I couldn't eat it as it is, but the capsules sound ok. I'll close my eyes and swallow it as if it was a vitamin," laughed Anita.

"Ok, I'll note here to keep the placenta for you. The hospital will wrap it up and store it until the person doing the encapsulation can come and get it. I know they need to pick it up within a certain period of time, but I'm not sure how long that is. You will have to ask once you contact them."

"I'll get onto it this afternoon."

"We'll add the name into your file at our next appointment, which will be in two weeks' time. The same day and time suit you?"

"Yes, thank you."

"That's it for today, then. Have a lovely rest of the day, Anita. And if anything happens or you have something to discuss, call or message me, ok? I'm here to support you."

Anita's eyes filled with tears again. "I am so happy to have you as my midwife. Thank you so much."

CHAPTER 24

The following few weeks sped by, with Anita's due day looming ahead. She had been enjoying the hypnobirthing classes and practicing it at night before falling asleep and in the morning after waking up. Sometimes, she even turned it on during the day when cleaning. It made the chore she didn't like a bit more bearable.

"Zara, I think the meditation is making a tremendous difference to my life. I'm not only preparing for the birth, I'm also more relaxed in my mind and body. I'm definitely going to continue with some sort of meditation after the baby is born as well. Are you finding it the same?" Anita asked Zara one day.

"Now you mention it, I am. I've been feeling quite stressed lately. We are rushing to finish the house before the baby comes and I'm still not over the morning sickness. It comes and goes, but I'm not as bad as you were," Zara added quickly. "Mine is mild, thank goodness. But yes, I have been all over the place and, well, how to say it nicely, harsh on Chris."

Anita giggled. "You mean you've been yelling at him?"

"Well, yes. Quite a lot," Zara admitted with a wink. "But the classes have been helping. I haven't been yelling as much; at least I don't think so. I wish I had the CD at home, but you need it more than I do right now, and I know that if I really wanted to, I could find something online. I just don't have time to search, and I can wait a few weeks. Chris will just have to endure me the way I am for now."

"I'm sure he's fine. Just blame it on the hormones; that's what I would do, anyway."

"Don't worry, that's what I've been doing. We'll see how long I get away with it. But you look amazing, Anita. You've now got the pregnancy glow I was telling you about."

"Do I? I can't see it, but I feel absolutely wonderful. That's true."

Anita had grown to love her changing body, cherishing her bump. Her pain had disappeared, as if by magic, two days after her third appointment. She woke up in the morning and walked to the loo as normal. After she sat on the toilet, it dawned on her.

"I'm not sore," she exclaimed. "I am not sore!" Her pubic bone hurt a little when peeing, but that was all; all the other pain had gone. A wide smile spread across her face. She felt amazing.

At the next osteopathy appointment, Anita told Lauren what had happened.

"How brilliant, Ms Wright. I'm so pleased with the progress you have made. I do recommend you to still continue with today's appointment, but if you are not sore, we won't book another one for now. If the pain comes back, you can always schedule more sessions later on. What do you think?"

"Yes, that sounds perfect," agreed Anita.

"Still, please continue doing the exercises I have given you at home. Don't stop doing those. They'll help you during delivery."

Anita's life had changed. She started going for long walks, enjoyed shopping trips, and even went to the movies; all the things she would have not dreamed of doing with the pain. A side effect of these outings was, however, people. *Why does a pregnant body have to attract so much attention?* Anita shuddered. *Where has this mentality come from?* Whenever she was out, someone rushed in to touch her belly and remark something awful or annoying. By someone, Anita meant women, especially the older generation.

"Oh my, look at you. You have little time left, don't you?" *Yes, but what's that to you?*

"I just have to touch your belly." *Um, no, you don't.*

"I'm sure it's a boy. I know it. I have the gift." *Well, you don't. You're wrong this time.*

"You are so big! Are you expecting twins?" *Nope. But thanks for pointing out how huge I have grown.*

"You poor little soul, giving birth is so painful. I'll be thinking of you." *Thank you for the encouragement. And you don't have to think of me. I don't even know you.*

All these well-meaning ladies made Anita furious. They made her so upset that now she rather crossed the road when she saw a woman approaching her. *Just keep your nose out of my business and leave me alone, will you?* At least her midwife understood, and they laughed about these ladies together.

"All pregnant women experience this at some level. It is a normal occurrence," said Josie.

"But why is it?" asked Anita. "They would never dare to walk to a woman who's not pregnant and touch her belly, or remark on her weight. So why, when a baby is involved, do they assume they can do so? I so want to tell them something back. Like 'Oh my, what an enormous head you've got' or 'It must be really hard to eat with teeth like that'. I know it sounds mean, but isn't it the same? Don't they know how unacceptable their behaviour is?"

"I don't think they do," said Josie. "In their own way, they are being nice and showing care."

"Well, somebody should tell them that they're not. At least I don't have long to go now, not long at all, and then this will all stop."

Anita groaned as a thought dawned on her. "But they will want to touch the baby when she's out, won't they?"

Josie nodded. "Yes, they probably will."

"Oh my, how do mothers do it? How do they deal with this unwanted attention to their child? I don't want strange women to ooh and ahh all over my baby and spit their germs on her."

"Yes, it is hard. We want to protect our children from the world, but the world wants them to be part of it. You'll have to find the balance that is comfortable for you. Never be afraid to tell people to back off. You are allowed to do so. This will be your child and you will be here to protect her or him. Don't listen to what people say; you will be the mother and nobody will ever care about your child's well-being as much as you. Nobody."

"Thank you, that's encouraging."

"Good. Now, let's check we've got all we need in place and listen to the baby. You've got only two weeks left. So, the baby could come any day now."

"Any day?" Anita gasped. "But I'm not ready."

"Well," smiled Josie, "the baby won't ask you. Don't dwell on the little things. You've got your birth plan, you've organised the placenta encapsulation, and you are practicing hypnobirthing. You are ready."

"I might be ready for the birth, but I don't have all the clothes I will need for the baby. I don't have the nursery set up properly and I don't have any meals pre-cooked. I still have so much to do."

"Have you packed the hospital bag for yourself and your baby?"

"Yes, I've done that."

"Good. Have you set up a safe sleeping space for the baby?"

"Yes, I've purchased a hammock. It's standing beside my bed now. I will keep the baby with me in my bedroom for the first few months."

"Perfect. Have you got some pads to use for bleeding after birth? You won't be able to use a cup for a while; it is not recommended and your vagina will need to contract again first."

"Not yet. I need to get those."

"Get them today, if possible. They'll give you a few at the hospital but, I imagine, you won't be sending the baby's father to buy you pads."

Anita's eyes grew wide. "No, you're right. That would not be appropriate. I can just imagine his face," Anita chortled. "It would be funny, but no, I'll rather get them myself."

"In regards to the baby's needs, as long as you have enough clothes and nappies for the baby to last you a week, you'll be fine. You've got a washing machine and the father can buy you more nappies."

"Oh, I've got plenty of nappies and I'll be using cloth later on. I've been shopping for such cute designs. You should see the fabrics they use. I can't wait to put them on the baby. And I've got some clothes already, enough to last me a week, I'm sure."

"Well, you've got all you need, then. Don't buy too much, babies grow so fast. I wouldn't worry much about the nursery; you can always finish it when the baby is here. She or he won't be interested in the world around for the first few weeks. Newborn babies don't see far either. All the baby will want to see is you."

"I can't wait for that. You always make me feel at such ease. Thank you."

"My pleasure. We'll book our last pregnancy appointment for the day before you're due. I'll then come to the birth, of course, and continue visiting you and the baby for a few months, too."

Josie entered it in her calendar and in Anita's book.

"Well now, let's listen to the baby's heartbeat and check how the baby is doing."

CHAPTER 25

"The baby is still turned the wrong way and is resting. I don't think anything is going to happen this weekend, Ms Wright."

At one o'clock on Friday afternoon, six days past her due date, Anita watched her baby sucking her thumb on the screen. Josie had asked her to have another scan to check on the baby's well-being.

"We have to check how the baby's doing. Most likely, it is comfortable inside you and not ready to come out yet. However, we need to know everything is ok, and the baby is not getting stressed. If nothing happens over the weekend, it will be the best to book your induction for Tuesday," said Josie.

Anita didn't want to be induced.

"Can we give the baby more time?"

"Well, we could wait for another few days, but I'm not sure if it's worth it. I wouldn't want the baby to become distressed. Your birthing experience would be much more challenging with a distressed baby."

"Ok," said Anita. "I will trust your experience, but I'm going to do whatever I can to get the baby moving."

"Good idea," said Josie. "Try going for long walks; exercise is supposed to help. Also, drinking raspberry leaf tea and eating spicy foods is said to work."

"Thank you, I'll give those a go."

Anita's efforts over the last two days had done little. The baby still enjoyed the comfort of her stomach and showed no signs of coming out. Although Anita loved seeing the baby on the screen, she would much rather hold her in her arms already.

"I will send the report to your midwife. I'm sure you've discussed a course of action, considering you are almost a week late now," said the sonographer while looking at her computer.

"Yes, we have. Thank you."

"Good luck, Ms Wright. Your baby is looking very healthy."

Anita walked back home, taking the longer route to get some extra exercise. She was barely noticing the beautiful day; too many worries cluttered her mind. She sighed in frustration.

So, after planning the perfect birth, I might need to be induced now? I don't want any drugs while the baby is inside me. I want the whole birth to be as natural as possible. Come on, baby! Come out already. I have waited for you for such a long time and I don't think I can wait any longer, Anita pleaded with her unborn.

At home, Anita tried to keep busy by organising the baby's room. She made a strong cup of raspberry leaf tea while snacking on spicy chips. *Yuck, how can people eat these? They are disgusting. You can't even taste what they actually taste like. They just burn your whole body; even my fingers are itchy now. I can't eat these,* she moaned and put the packet aside.

Oh, I'm leaking again.

Anita had had some vaginal discharge during her pregnancy, especially now towards the end. She walked to the loo to clean herself.

"Well, this is different," she said after pulling her knickers down, staring at the, for the lack of a better word, blob. Not like her usual discharge, this had blood strewn through and was of a much thicker consistency.

Maybe something is happening.

At three o'clock, only two hours after her scan, the first contraction arrived. The intensity and suddenness of it bent Anita forward.

Well, something is definitely happening, gasped Anita.

"Zara, I think I'm having contractions," she said when Zara picked up the phone.

"You are? How exciting! I'll come straight away to take you to the hospital."

"Hold on, I don't think you have to come right now; it's still too early. Apparently, it can take a few hours or sometimes a few days for the baby to arrive, but I hope it doesn't take that long. I've only had one, if that was it, but it couldn't have been anything else, right?"

"I imagine you can't mistake a contraction. Have you recorded the time and length?"

"Oh no, I didn't. I forgot about the app I downloaded. I'll record the next one and call you when it's time for hospital, ok?"

"Perfect. I'm still helping Grandpa, but if you need me, I can leave."

"Thank you."

Anita searched for the app she had downloaded. *Ok, I'll record the next one.*

She didn't have to wait long; the next wave came soon

after. Anita pressed the button at the beginning, crumpling down onto the sofa in the kitchen. She found it easier to deal with the pain in a horizontal position. As suddenly as it came on, it was over.

Only 34 seconds. That can't be too serious yet. I need to let George know.

She had almost forgotten about George. "George, I'm in labour."

"You are? I'm coming over," blurted George.

"No, don't come. It could take several hours or days before anything happens. I'll let you know when Zara takes me to the hospital."

"Ok. I will come with you straight away."

"But I could be in the hospital for days."

"I don't mind. I'm coming with you. I want to be there when the baby is born."

"Not in the room!"

George laughed with relief in his voice. "No, not in the room. That would be weird for both of us, wouldn't it? And my stomach might not agree with it either."

"Good. I'll be in touch."

The next contraction came about 12 minutes after the second one, with more strength this time. Anita curled up on the sofa, waiting for it to stop. Sitting at 39 seconds, it was still short. The following one arrived earlier, only 6 minutes later, finishing at 44 seconds, but the one after didn't come until almost 4pm and lasted only 20 seconds. Anita wasn't sure what to make out of the times.

Zara rushed into the house at 4.30, while Anita lay curled up with yet another contraction, the third one since the short one half an hour prior. The contractions were getting more frequent and longer, but Anita had expected them to be much stronger; she had expected unbearable pain. This wasn't at all what she had read about. This pain was weaker than what she had experienced with her pelvis pain.

"Were you having a nap?" said Zara with a grin after she located Anita.

"I wish. I was having another contraction."

"I couldn't stay away. I'll rather wait here with you. How are you going?" said Zara with concern.

"Going."

Another wave announced its arrival.

"It's here again," she gasped and suffered through it. "Uff, this one was strong. And I didn't record it. It's so hard to record them while having them."

"Never fear, I'm here now and I'll be the official contraction recorder," said Zara in an official sounding voice.

Anita pleaded, "Can you also be the tea brewing specialist? I've got a box of raspberry leaf tea in the cupboard; it's supposed to bring labour on."

"So, I shouldn't make one for myself?"

"I don't suppose it would work when you're still in the first trimester, but you never know."

"Hmm, I won't risk it. I'll have a nice mint tea instead. A nice cuppa will do me good. I've been so gassy lately. Pregnancy throws your whole body off, doesn't it? What it does to you is unbelievable, and nobody can really prepare you for it."

"Yep, I agree."

"Zara! A contraction," cried Anita.

Zara grabbed Anita's phone. "Oh, I don't know your lock combination. Bugger. I can't record it."

"Thank goodness this one is over," Anita winced. "They're not as bad as I had expected, but still."

"That's good, but I failed at the recording. I couldn't get into your phone. It started at 4:41 and lasted less than a minute, for sure. The time didn't jump to the next minute during it," said Zara. "You know what? I'll download the app and record them on my phone."

Zara concentrated on her phone for a minute. "I'm ready now. Come, have another one. I want to try it," giggled Zara.

"It's not funny," groaned Anita.

"I know, sorry. I'm just so excited."

Zara's wish came true a minute later.

"It's here," called Anita, curling up on the corner sofa.

"4:48 and 43 seconds."

"4:53 and 31 seconds."

"5:04 and 54 seconds."

"5:09 and 36 seconds."

"5:16 and 51 seconds."

"Anita, we should call the midwife. You are in a lot of pain."

"But the contractions are not five minutes apart and lasting about a minute. They are all over the place," disagreed Anita.

"I don't care what the times say, you must be further along than you think. Give me the number and I'll call her; better to check with her, don't you think?"

Anita had just enough time to unlock her phone when another contraction arrived.

"5:21 and 50 seconds."

"I'm calling her now," said Zara.

Anita didn't even register Zara talking. She was busy waiting for another contraction.

"She said to come to the hospital now."

"Oh, ok. Can you let George know? He wants to come with us."

Zara called George. "Ok, he knows and will meet us there. Come up now. I'll help you into the car."

As Anita clambered to her feet, another contraction came. And, possibly with the help of gravity, her water broke at the same time.

Warm stream gushed down Anita's legs and all over the kitchen floor.

"My water broke."

"Your water broke," said Zara at the same time.

"I'll grab some towels." Zara sprinted upstairs to the cupboard.

Anita stared at the amount of water on the floor. She caused a complete flood. What alarmed her, however, was the colour. It should have been clear, but had a green tinge to it. "Zara, the water's not clear. Quick!"

Zara rushed into the room; hands full of towels. "Everything is ok, you'll see," said Zara, trying to calm Anita down as she spread some towels on the floor. She gave the rest to Anita. "We'll take these into the car for you to sit on. I can't have you messing up my car," she chuckled.

"You should grab a plastic sheet then or tie me to the roof," grumped Anita.

"Sorry, I'm not trying to upset you. I thought a joke would help. Obviously not."

"Actually, Zara, I still have some of the pants you brought for my miscarriage. They're in the drawer in the upstairs bathroom. Can you grab one?"

"Great idea. I'll be right back." Zara returned in a jiffy.

"Here you go. Put them on. Ok, where are your hospital bags?"

"By the door," said Anita, while putting the incontinence pants on.

Zara ran outside with the bags.

"Got them. Are you ready?"

Zara pushed Anita out of the house and into the car, arranging a pile of towels underneath her. Running to the driver's side, she jumped in and sped off. Another contraction came, and a gush of water followed. Anita saw Zara glancing at her.

"I'm ok, don't rush. You're driving like a madman."

"Yes, I know. I want to get you to the hospital."

Parking in front of the hospital, Zara jumped out and ran

inside. Anita clambered out of the car and, holding onto the car first, made the few steps to the hospital wall.

"Why didn't you wait in the car?" exclaimed Zara, rushing towards her.

A nurse with a wheelchair appeared behind her. "Sit down please, madam. I'll take you inside."

"I'll park the car and come," Anita heard Zara calling, but she was lost in another contraction.

"Good evening, Anita. How are you doing?" Josie greeted Anita as the nurse wheeled her into the birthing room.

"Oh, you're already here," said Anita in surprise. "That's good. I'm doing, I guess. I've just finished another contraction."

"Yes, I was at the hospital when your friend called. Can you talk me through what has happened so far?"

"My contractions are all over the place. They are sporadic, from a few minutes apart to 10 plus minutes, neither of them longer than a minute. Some are strong, some are not; and my water broke."

"Your water broke? When?"

"Before coming here. I stood up and had a contraction at the same time, and it all went. Lucky I was in the kitchen and nowhere with a carpet, but the water had a greenish tinge to it."

"I'm afraid you cannot do water birth, Anita. The colour means the baby has relieved into the water. Most likely, it is because you are past your due date and the baby just couldn't hold it any longer, but it might also mean the baby is stressed. We'll have to put electrodes on the baby's head for monitoring."

Anita only nodded, feeling another contraction coming

on. The last thing she heard was a nurse telling someone to stop running the water. She leaned on the bed, waiting for it to stop.

"I need to see how far along you are," Josie said when the contraction had finished.

A nurse helped Anita to lie on the bed. They stripped the incontinence pants off.

"This was a good idea," Josie said, examining the colour inside.

"I had some left at home from my miscarriage. I didn't want to gush water all over my friend's car." Anita grinned, "Although she still made me sit on a pile of towels."

"You were right to come in, Anita. You are fully dilated and with the next contraction, can start pushing."

Anita's mouth dropped open. "I'm ready? The baby is coming? Like now? Shouldn't it take several hours for anything to happen? I've been having contractions only since three. Even the sonographer said that nothing was happening this weekend because the baby was so calm."

"Well, your baby is obviously not listening to the sonographer or the material you have read, and is coming now."

Anita felt another contraction coming on. "It's here," she said before the cramps hit.

"Push as hard as you can, Anita," said Josie.

Anita tried, but nothing much happened. So, when the contraction had finished and Josie said, "I can see the head. Hold still please while I attach the electrodes," Anita gasped in surprise.

She's coming. My baby is coming, she rejoiced.

With Josie busy between her legs, Anita had a revelation.

Yet again, I have someone looking at my intimate parts, but at this moment, I don't care. I just want the baby to be out of me.

"All done."

"Can I turn around and kneel? I heard gravity can help."

"Yes, certainly. Here, let the nurse help you."

A nurse supported Anita to turn while Josie adjusted the bed.

"Are you comfortable?"

Anita kneeled, holding onto the head of the bed, which Josie had raised straight upwards. "Yes, this is better."

Anita gasped as another wave hit her.

"Push, Anita. Push," Josie called.

And Anita pushed with all her might.

Oh, how it burns. Why does it feel like my vagina is burning? Am I on fire? Spray me with water, someone, just spray me with water.

"Continue pushing, Anita. You don't have to wait for another contraction. Just push, the baby is coming."

Anita pushed. She didn't breathe; in the commotion forgetting her hypnobirthing training. The day had been like a rollercoaster, but she needed to calm down and bring this baby into the world. Gathering the rest of the composure she had left, Anita drew air in, inhaling and exhaling in rhythm, soothing her whole body. With every exhale, she pushed with all the strength she had left.

"The head is out. You're almost finished."

Another exhale and Anita pushed. The burning sensation had stopped, a surge of movement followed, and finally the feeling of release filled her body.

"The baby is here. You are all done, Anita."

The nurse helped Anita to turn onto her back. They lowered the bed before placing the newborn onto her chest.

"Let me help you pull the top of your dress down. Skin to skin is critical in the first days, especially straight after birth."

Anita looked into the little, wrinkled face in her arms. The baby was still dirty from her womb, but she was already the most beautiful thing she had ever seen.

"Your baby is a girl, Anita." Josie confirmed what Anita had always known.

"She's perfect. Aren't you little one? You are perfect."

Anita caressed her baby, loving her already more than anything else in the universe, her heart stretching and bursting so much she worried it might pop like an over-inflated balloon.

"See if she latches on. She might be hungry."

Anita gave it a go. Supported by Josie, she offered her infant her nipple; and she latched on almost immediately. "She was hungry," Anita gasped.

Her baby slurped and sucked the milk and Anita watched, enjoying the odd but beautiful sensation.

"Would you like to cut the cord?" Josie asked. "We've delayed it enough; all the nutrients have gone through now.

"Yes, please."

A nurse passed Anita a serrated pair of scissors and showed her where to cut in between two clamps. She struggled to cut through while holding the baby, but at the end managed.

"Do you want to keep some of the cord?"

"I do, thanks."

Anita returned her attention to the baby still attached to her breast. Her eyes were shut, and she was suckling with power.

"Anita, I'm sorry to interrupt this moment, but you'll need to start pushing again to get the placenta out now."

Anita pushed and pushed, but nothing much happened.

"Do you want to try on the loo? It might work better. I'll give you a bowl and while you are trying, I'll clean the baby and measure her."

Anita reluctantly passed her little girl to Josie. A nurse supported her to the bathroom; in her exhausted state, the few steps felt miles away.

"Here's a bowl for the placenta, a towel, and a hospital

gown. You will feel better after having a shower and getting out of your soiled dress. Call if you need anything."

Anita grabbed everything and walked into the bathroom. The droplets of warm water falling on her body quenched some of the weariness and pain. Putting the bowl on the toilet seat, she tried to push into it. Nothing happened. Straining a few more times with the same result, she got dressed and returned to the room.

Josie was bending over her baby, measuring her head. "She's perfect, Anita," she said. "Exactly as she should be. You've got a beautiful baby girl."

"I know she is," said Anita in response, her heart bursting at seams.

"I'm afraid the placenta didn't come out."

"Ok, can you lie down on the bed again, please? I will give you your baby and we'll try to pull it out."

Anita settled down with her daughter in her arms. She pulled down the hospital gown to allow skin to skin again.

"I will try to pull on the cord and you push Anita, ok?"

"Ok."

Anita pushed and pushed until her strength and will to continue depleted.

"I'm afraid the cord has snapped. You seem to have retained placenta."

"What does it mean?"

"It means it's likely attached to the uterus wall and will need to be surgically removed."

"Like now?"

"Yes, we will have to take you to the theatre now. You'll go under anaesthesia and the surgeon will take the placenta out."

"But what about my baby? She cannot be without me for so long."

"She will be ok," Josie assured Anita. "Your friend is waiting outside, isn't she? We will invite her in and she can wait with your daughter until your surgery is finished and you wake up again."

Anita resisted that idea. She just had her baby and now they were going to take her away from her? She didn't want that. This couldn't be happening! Anita's eyes welled with tears.

"I know it's not ideal, but everything will be ok and you will see your baby soon. It has to be done, Anita. The placenta needs to come out."

"Ok, if it's the last resort, then I have to do it."

"Good. But first, while you are giving her another little suck, do you have a name for her? You don't have to but if you do, I'll write it in the documentation already."

"I have. Her name is Ella."

"Beautiful. It fits her well. She looks like Ella," said Josie and wrote it into her notes. "And so you know, Ella was born at 19:19. Such a great time."

Anita smiled at her from the bed.

"Ok, do you want to cover your body? I'll invite your friend in and you can tell her what's happening."

"Ella's father, George, should be there too. He can also come in."

Josie walked to the door. "Are you Zara and George? You can come in now."

The two rushed in like an avalanche and crowded around Anita, admiring the baby.

"Oh my goodness, look at the baby. How beautiful. Is it a girl?" Zara blurted out.

"Hello, you two. Meet Ella."

Anita's heart was bursting with pride and love.

"She's perfect, isn't she?"

"She is. Can I hold her?" George couldn't take his eyes off his baby daughter.

"Yes, you can. You will actually have to look after her for me for a while. My placenta hasn't come out, so they need to take me to the theatre to remove it. You two will have to stay with Ella."

"Oh, are you ok?"

Zara's and George's eyes showed genuine concern.

"Yes, I am. It wasn't as bad as I had expected, and the surgery has to be done. I'm not happy about it, but ..." Anita shrugged her shoulders. She wished she felt as calm inside as she pretended to be on the outside.

"Are you ready, Anita? It's time," said Josie.

"Yes, I am. I'll see you soon, little one." Anita passed the baby to George.

"Look after her as if she was your own," she added, winking.

George smiled at her. "I will. I will protect her like a lion."

The nurse wheeled Anita's bed out of the room. The last thing she saw was George holding her beautiful baby and Zara fussing over her. Her eyes filled with tears; the turmoil inside her making its way out. She didn't see the hallways the nurse was pushing her through. Her vision blurred with bitter tears and her heart aching, Anita lost the battle with her mind.

CHAPTER 26

Anita woke up. She stared at the ceiling, trying to remember where she was. Then her mind clicked, and she sat up with a jerk, her heart running wild. A wave of relief and happiness washed over her body when she saw her newborn in a see-through crib beside her bed. Leaning over, she admired the tiny face and hands peeking out of the bundle.

"You're awake. Good."

Anita looked up to find George sitting in an armchair across the room.

"Hello," said Anita. At least she attempted to, but nothing much came out. Her voice was hoarse and almost non-existent.

"Here, have some water." George strode to her bed, passing her a glass.

"Thank you."

"How beautiful is she?" George said, looking at his

daughter with so much love that Anita's heart swelled. Tears rolled down her cheeks and her whole body filled with warmth she hadn't experienced before.

"She is perfect," whispered Anita, her eyes locking with George's. "We did a great job."

"Yes, we did. But you did all the work. I'm glad the birth went well."

"Yes, it went very well; I'm relieved, trust me. I've read of some horror experiences. Did you know that some women spend two days in painful labour and still have to have a c-section? I can't even imagine going through that. Even my contractions were not that awful."

"Good evening, Ms Wright," a nurse, walking into the room, said. "How are you feeling?"

"I guess ok. Still sore, and my voice has gone," she rasped.

"That's normal after anaesthesia, it will come back soon. Have you been to the loo?"

"No, I've just woken up."

"Can you please go and try now? It will be uncomfortable at the beginning, but we need to know it all works. And I'll get you some food in the meantime. You are hungry, aren't you?"

Anita's stomach rumbled at the mention of food. "Yes, I'm hungry."

"Come, I'll show you where the bathroom is. Here's a towel if you want to wash."

Anita slunk off the bed and limped towards the door.

"Your midwife has gone home but will be back in the morning. Your placenta is wrapped up and stored in the fridge, and your midwife has organised the placenta encapsulation person to come and pick it up tomorrow."

"Oh, she has? Wonderful. She's the best."

During the eventful evening, Anita had completely forgotten about the encapsulation service.

"Here's the bathroom, and I'll be back soon with your food," said the nurse, hurrying off.

Anita sat on the loo and hissed in pain. It burned so much that she had to stop. *I'll have a shower first and try again,* she thought.

She washed all the sweat off, washing some of her troubles off as well. Then she sat on the toilet again. It burned and stung too much for Anita to even dare to push harder. *What if it hurts even more? I can't do this. I don't really need to go, anyway. It will work soon enough, I'm sure.*

With Ella still asleep, Anita crawled back into bed. A tray awaited her on the hospital table. The nurse had brought her a large cup of tea, two sandwiches, a banana, a muffin, a pot of yoghurt, and a small tub of ice cream. Anita pulled the table towards her, eating with relish.

George watched her, amused. "You were hungry."

"Starving."

Ella's little eyes opened. Anita pushed the table away, almost tipping the tea over in her rush to get to her daughter.

"Hello beautiful. How are you doing? Would you like to come up to your mummy?" Anita said, picking Ella up, her heart aching.

How can such a little person bring on so much love?

Ella settled into Anita's arms in a natural embrace, her little eyes gazing into Anita's face. They were meant for each other; they were perfect together.

Ella wriggled, grizzling.

"Oh, you can talk, can you? I haven't heard you yet."

The grizzle turned into a more intense cry.

Anita laughed, "You surely can. Are you hungry? Would you like some milk?" Anita brought the baby to her chest. Ella knew what to do and latched on straight away. "You were hungry. Look at you. We will be great together, won't we?"

Anita did not know if Ella latched on well. Neither of them had any experience, but in Anita's elated state, she didn't care. She watched Ella's little eyes closing and opening, her mouth moving in rhythm with her sucking, and listened to her swallowing the milk. When Ella released Anita's nipple, she grizzled again.

"Oh, are you still hungry? I can give you some more from the other side. Shall we try?" Anita moved Ella to her other breast where she continued her feed until she unlatched, her tummy full.

Anita gazed into Ella's face when George said, "Can I hold her please? I'll have to go home now; I've got a private lesson in the morning."

Anita looked up in alarm. She had forgotten about George, who watched her giving Ella milk. Oh no, she had both her breasts out.

"Yes, you can." Anita's cheeks turned bright red.

George guessed he had made her uncomfortable. "You don't have to be embarrassed. It was beautiful."

This made Anita turn crimson. She passed Ella to George and covered herself with a blanket. Feeding in public was definitely not her thing.

"Goodbye, Ella, I'll come back tomorrow. Sleep well." George kissed Ella's forehead and gave her back to Anita.

"I'll see you in the morning, Anita. Try to rest."

"Good night, George. Thank you for being here."

"You're welcome. I wouldn't want to be anywhere else."

Anita caressed Ella's head and face, trying to imprint the little details into her memory. She knew George was watching them, but she had someone much more important in her arms to care. Finally, the door had closed behind George.

"It's only the two of us now, my beautiful."

Ella closed her eyes.

"Are you sleepy again? You must be. Being born is a

tiring experience, isn't it? You've done a great job coming out so fast. Thank you."

But Ella had closed her eyes already.

"Sleep well, my little one. I'll put you back into your cot, ok? I'll try to sleep as well."

Anita lowered Ella back into the cot, wrapping her up in a warm blanket. Ella grizzled after leaving the warmth of Anita's embrace, but settled almost instantly. Anita laid back down on the bed, watching the tiny bundle. *How perfect could one little person be?*

Anita's own attempts at falling asleep proved fruitless. Ella's irregular breathing kept her wide awake. She gasped and often didn't take another breath for a few seconds. Anita had read newborns take a little while to settle into a normal breathing rhythm, but she had never expected this. No way will she get any sleep when she was too scared to even close her eyes.

What if Ella stops breathing when I sleep? ... Oh no, I didn't burp her after the feed. What if she spews and then chokes on it? How do mothers even function? I can't imagine doing anything else than keeping her safe. Oh no, is this what motherhood is about? Constantly worrying and fretting? ... But she's so beautiful. We'll be fine. We have to be! It's all good, she's ok and I'm ok and we will be great together. If something was wrong with her lungs, they would have picked up on it already, wouldn't they? ... Aargh, I need to get some sleep. I'm exhausted. How am I going to function tomorrow? ... Stop thinking; stop thinking and close your eyes. Ella is fine. She is healthy and sleeping, and I need to sleep, too.

Anita wanted to quieten her thoughts, but her mind raced from one terrible scenario to another. Eventually, she fell into an uneasy sleep.

"Good morning, Ms Wright," said the nurse.

Anita woke up in alarm, turning to Ella, who was still sleeping.

"Here's your breakfast. Did you get some sleep?"

"I guess I did," Anita said. "I didn't think I would, but I must have. I couldn't stop looking at the baby. Her breathing is so irregular and I had to listen to it, in case something went wrong, you know?"

"You're not the only one. It takes some time to get used to having a little human beside you. The breathing will stabilise soon. It's normal."

"Yes, so I've read, but it's still alarming."

"She's well and healthy, you don't have to worry. Your midwife will talk to you more about her soon. You just need to stop stressing and sleep whenever she sleeps. You will need it."

"Well, how encouraging," Anita said to herself after the nurse had left. "You will need it, she said." Anita whimpered, "What have we got ourselves into, my princess? What have we got ourselves into?"

During breakfast, Josie walked in. "Good morning, Anita. How was your first night as a mother?"

"Good morning. It was great. Tiring, but amazing."

"I hope you got some sleep."

"Yes, I did; only after watching Ella for hours, fretting about her breathing."

Josie smiled. "That was to be expected. You'll get used to her being with you soon, but try to sleep as much as possible today. The second night tends to be hard with Ella probably wanting to feed a lot. Not because she'll hungry, rather for comfort. She'll soon figure out that you are here for her and that she feels the most comfortable in your arms. And so, she will want to be with you all the time. Some babies don't do it, but most do, so be prepared for a sleepless night."

Anita chuckled, "So that's what the nurse must have meant this morning. She told me to sleep today because I will need it."

"Yes, the nurses know. They've seen it all. How are you otherwise? Have you been to the loo?"

"No, I haven't. I tried last night but I couldn't do it. It hurt too much."

"Can you go now, please? We need to make sure everything is fine. Holding urine is bad for your bladder and birth can mess things up. You will not have a bowel movement for another day or two, but urine needs to be passed."

Anita shuffled out the door to the bathroom. Sitting on the toilet, she pushed. Relieved the pain had subsided, she urinated.

They say giving birth is an ordeal, but nobody mentions what happens afterwards. This is the hard part, the after-birth time, thought Anita.

"All good?" asked Josie when she had returned to her room.

"Yes, I did pee."

"Perfect. Ella is waking up so I'll check on her and while you feed her, I'll correct your latch, if necessary. And if everything goes well, you'll be able to go home midday tomorrow, if you like."

Anita beamed at the prospect.

Her first day as a mother flew by. Zara and George arrived pretty much at the same time and stayed almost forever. Anita didn't want to send them away, but all she had wanted was to have some alone time with her baby and try to sleep. When the night came, she could barely hold her eyes open.

Anita was emotionally prepared for the night, but it still came with a shock. Ella wanted to be held almost constantly, trying to suck and screaming her head off when not sucking.

Anita spent half of the night walking with her in her arms and the other half feeding her. At four in the morning, a nurse walked in.

"Have you had any sleep, Ms Wright?"

Anita shook her head.

"Here, let me take her and you get some sleep."

"But she needs me. She needs milk," said Anita, not wanting to give her Ella.

"She will be ok, trust me. She needs you well rested. I'll take her with me and you get some sleep."

Anita passed Ella over with reluctance. The nurse put her into the cot and wheeled the cot out of the room. With her baby gone, Anita burst into tears.

Get a grip on yourself, you silly. Ella is safe. Lie down and get some sleep.

Anita collapsed on the bed, absolutely exhausted. Without Ella in the room, she dropped into a deep sleep almost instantly.

Where am I? Anita woke up in confusion. The sun streamed into the window; a bird sang in the distance and a baby cried in the neighbouring room.

"Ella! Where is Ella?" Anita almost ran out of the door into the nurses' room.

"Good morning, Ms Wright. Did you have a sleep?" a nurse welcomed her.

"I did, yes. Where is Ella?"

"She's here. She's had a good sleep too." The nurse pointed at the cot behind her where Ella slept peacefully.

"You don't need to worry. We've looked after her well for you."

"Thank you. Can I take her back to my room now?"

"I'll bring her in for you."

The nurse wheeled the cot back to Anita's room, with Anita following closely. In her deep sleep, Ella didn't even stir.

"Here you are. I'll bring you your breakfast."

Anita's full attention returned to her baby. She was so beautiful, just perfect. Yet again, her heart swelled so much it almost burst.

"So, this is love. I love you so much, little one," she whispered, staring at her daughter.

Josie walked in about 30 minutes later. "Good morning, Anita. I heard you both got some sleep last night."

"We did, and we're both much better for it," said Anita, sitting on the bed with Ella in her arms.

"Ella has just woken up," she said in explanation before offering Ella her nipple. Ella latched on, gulping her milk. "She is starving."

"A good sleep would do that," said Josie. "You can go home soon, if you like. Or you can stay one more night. You had a surgery, so the choice is yours."

"I want to go home, please."

"I thought you would. I'll get the nurse to check your vitals and the doctor will discharge you. You could be ready in about an hour."

Anita looked up in surprise. "So soon?"

"Yes," laughed Josie. "No need to keep you here longer than necessary."

"Wonderful. I'll call Zara to bring the car seat and come to pick us up."

"Do. And I'll get the nurse to do the paperwork."

Josie left Anita alone.

"We're going home, my pretty girl."

During the next hour, several people came and went, until Anita had the discharge papers in her hands. After getting changed into her normal clothes and packing their bags, she picked Ella out of the cot.

Zara burst into the room. "Good day to you two. Are you ready?"

"Yes, more than ready."

Zara grabbed Anita's bags, excited as much as Anita herself. "I'm as happy as if it was me," she said. "Come on, ladies. I'll take you home."

Anita thanked all the nurses as they walked past their room. Clutching the precious bundle in her arms, she stepped into the bright day outside. The sun welcomed them, caressing their cheeks with its warmth. Anita accepted it as a sign, a sign from Mother Nature. Anita's life had taken the happiest turn. She had become a mother. Her dream had come true.

The End?

Well, no. Rather the Beginning.

Now you have finished my book, I would really appreciate you leaving a review.

Reviews are the best rewards for us authors as they allow us to understand what our readers want and how they feel and by that support us in writing better books in the future.

Please, scan this review QR code

And if you want to keep in touch with my world of writing and be the first to know about new releases, sales, and events, please sign up to my newsletter on my website www.ivetaongley.com And don't forget to claim your FREE pdf downloads.

ABOUT THE AUTHOR

Iveta Ongley is a Czech Kiwi author and teacher living in New Zealand.
She is the author of several children's picture and chapter books. Out of the norm is her first novel for adult audience.

When she's not writing, she can be found scouring the stunning local beaches for shells, listening to birdsong in the bush, and catching up on some well-deserved sleep. With two kids and two cats by her side, and a husband, who all keep her busy, she's never short on inspiration. What she's short on is time to put all the creative ideas spinning in her head on paper. Her biggest wish is to be able to clone herself.

www.ingramcontent.com/pod-product-compliance
Lightning Source LLC
Chambersburg PA
CBHW031106080526
44587CB00011B/854